TABLE OF CONTENTS

Top 20 Test Taking Tips

1. Carefully follow all the test registration procedures
2. Know the test directions, duration, topics, question types, how many questions
3. Setup a flexible study schedule at least 3-4 weeks before test day
4. Study during the time of day you are most alert, relaxed, and stress free
5. Maximize your learning style; visual learner use visual study aids, auditory learner use auditory study aids
6. Focus on your weakest knowledge base
7. Find a study partner to review with and help clarify questions
8. Practice, practice, practice
9. Get a good night's sleep; don't try to cram the night before the test
10. Eat a well balanced meal
11. Know the exact physical location of the testing site; drive the route to the site prior to test day
12. Bring a set of ear plugs; the testing center could be noisy
13. Wear comfortable, loose fitting, layered clothing to the testing center; prepare for it to be either cold or hot during the test
14. Bring at least 2 current forms of ID to the testing center
15. Arrive to the test early; be prepared to wait and be patient
16. Eliminate the obviously wrong answer choices, then guess the first remaining choice
17. Pace yourself; don't rush, but keep working and move on if you get stuck
18. Maintain a positive attitude even if the test is going poorly
19. Keep your first answer unless you are positive it is wrong
20. Check your work, don't make a careless mistake

Score Reporting

Use the following link: for the most information about score reporting:
http://www.nursingworld.org/ancc/certification/cert/exams/NewRptFormat.html

Be Aware of the Following

1. Currently the exam is a 175-question test that covers all of the content listed in the following link:
   http://www.nursingworld.org/ancc/certification/cert/exams/TCOs/ACNPTCO.html
2. Only 150 questions count toward your test score.
3. The exams are offered primarily on computer year round and with paper/pencil on occasion.
4. Make sure you are registered for the exam. Go to: http://www.nursingworld.org/ancc/ to register.
5. Review the handbook offered by the ANCC for the test you are taking.
6. Take the practice questions offered by the ANCC for the test you are taking.

Assessment of Acute and Chronic Illness

Epidemiology and Disease Control

Epidemiology

Epidemiology is defined as the study of the occurrence, frequency, and distribution of disease within a population. This is a rather broad definition, however, and the field of epidemiology encompasses far more than the definition suggests. Many clinicians are removed from epidemiological research in daily practice, and are far more affected by advances in epidemiology than they may realize. Epidemiology includes the study of biological, social, and environmental factors as they relate to the spread of disease within and across populations and communities in an effort to understand, control, and treat the diseases that affect our patients and ourselves. It is important, then, for clinicians to be aware of the benefits of epidemiological study, and to become active participants in the prevention of disease.

Use in nursing field

Epidemiology is important to nurses across all clinical settings, not just those in public health positions. Each and every nurse will treat a varied patient population during his or her career, and it is important for the nurse to create a plan of care that is tailored to the patient; the patient's age, race, career, and religion all represent different populations to which he or she belongs, and may affect clinical course, treatment, and outcome. Armed with epidemiological knowledge about his or her patients, the nurse can create a clinical decision-making framework, an effective care plan, and the means to share this information with his or her peers to aid in the care of other patients.

Pathophysiology

Cardiovascular

Hypertension

Primary hypertension is a somewhat complicated disease state that has no known single cause, but rather a constellation of contributing factors. The presence and interaction of these various factors will vary from patient to patient, and, as such, a detailed history and physical examination are necessary. Some patients with primary hypertension demonstrate either a defect in sodium excretion or the inability to regulate angiotensin II, attributing the pathogenesis of the hypertension to the kidneys and/or adrenal glands. An increase in activity of the sympathetic nervous system is also attributed to primary hypertension, either through chronically elevated epinephrine or dysfunction of the sympathetic baroreceptors, which cause prolonged increases in vascular resistance. A decrease in nitric oxide (which is the most potent vasodilator produced by the body) also may contribute to the pathogenesis of primary hypertension.

Left ventricular hypertrophy:
Longstanding primary hypertension will eventually take a toll on other organs in the body, perhaps the heart most of all. Left ventricular hypertrophy is the most common complication of longstanding primary hypertension involving the heart. Left ventricular hypertrophy (LVH) is a thickening of the muscular wall (myocardium) of the left ventricle in response to increased pressure in the aorta, as well as increased peripheral vascular resistance. The high pressure in the aorta and other arteries means that the left ventricle must pump harder to overcome that resistance and move the blood into the arteries; the higher the blood pressure, and the longer the pressure is elevated, the harder the left ventricle will have to work, and the thicker the myocardium will become.

Hypertrophic Cardiomyopathy

Hypertrophic cardiomyopathy is a disease in which the size (thickness) of the cardiac muscle is increased. In some patients this is due to an outflow tract obstruction, and in others it is idiopathic (meaning that the cause is unknown). In most cases of hypertrophic cardiomyopathy, however, the individual will have an enlarged left ventricle in addition to the enlarged muscle itself. Individuals will usually have some degree of septal enlargement as well. The enlarged left ventricle leads to an increase in the volume and the pressure in the left ventricle, as well as an increase in the volume and the pressure of the left atrium.

Congenital Defects

Aortic valve:
The aortic valve may be stenotic, meaning that the valve opening does not widen as much as it should, making the valve more narrow, which in turn makes it more difficult for the blood to flow through. Aortic stenosis may result in congestive heart failure, syncope, dizziness, and angina. The aortic valve may also be insufficient, meaning that it does not function properly, allowing blood to leak backwards during ventricular diastole. Also, a third leaflet may fail to form, which is called "bicuspid aortic valve." Individuals with a bicuspid aortic valve may not have any symptoms early on, though they are at greater risk of certain complications later in life, including calcifications of the valve leaflets (leading to stenosis and/or regurgitation) and aortic dissection.

Arrhythmias

An arrhythmia is a condition in which the heart beats abnormally; there are many different causes of arrhythmia, and the majority of them are benign. An arrhythmia can either be supraventricular, meaning that it begins in the atria, or it can be ventricular, originating in the ventricles. Arrhythmias are further classified by heart rate; a heart rate below 60 beats per minute is called bradycardia, and a rate above 100 bpm is called tachycardia. Tachycardia that is uncoordinated is called fibrillation, and is much more serious. Symptoms of arrhythmia include palpitations or "skipped beats," fatigue, shortness of breath (dyspnea), light-headedness, and chest pain. In addition, a patient with tachycardia may be sweaty and dizzy.

Vasculitis

Vasculitis is a syndrome in which the walls of the blood vessels become inflamed, causing a disruption of blood flow and resulting in either transient or prolonged ischemia. The most common vasculitis is giant-cell arteritis (GCA) (sometimes called temporal arteritis, because the temporal artery is commonly, but not uniquely, involved); the disease is characterized by a mononuclear infiltrate of lymphocytes and plasma cells that form into giant cells containing multiple nuclei. Large- and medium-sized arteries are affected by GCA. Polyarteritis nodosa (PAN), on the other hand, involves medium and small arteries, and is characterized by an infiltrate of neutrophils. The neutrophils degranulate, causing focal, segmental necrosis of the vessels and surrounding tissue. Henoch-Schönlein purpura is also a necrotizing vasculitis similar to PAN, though it occurs mostly in children, and is limited to the skin, small and large bowel, and kidneys.

Pulmonary

Acute Respiratory Distress Syndrome

Adult respiratory distress syndrome (ARDS) is a result of the pulmonary response to shock. Whether a shock patient will develop ARDS, and the severity of the lung injury, depends on a number of factors, including the severity of the shock, as well as whether the patient has any other preexisting lung disease or damage. The hallmark characteristic of ARDS is a decrease in lung compliance. The decrease in compliance is a result of massive pulmonary edema in the absence of increased left atrial pressure. The interstitial edema compresses pulmonary blood flow, resulting in shunting, and, ultimately, hypoxia. The hypoxia is compounded by the decrease in lung compliance, because inspiratory volume is severely limited.

Airflow Obstruction

The 5 mechanisms by which airflow can be compromised and/or obstructed include expiratory airway collapse, bronchospasm, mucosal inflammation and edema, mucinous gland hypertrophy, and external compression of the airway.

- Expiratory airway collapse occurs in patients with loss of rigidity of the cartilage backbone of the airways. As air is forced out of the airways during expiration, the softened cartilage can no longer hold the airways open, and they collapse in on themselves. Symptoms of expiratory airway collapse mimic asthma and chronic obstructive pulmonary disease (COPD), but although they may have similar presentations, the mechanisms are different. The softening of cartilage that leads to expiratory airway collapse is called tracheobronchomalacia. Expiratory airway collapse can also be caused by excessive dynamic airway collapse (EDAC), which is due not to softening of the cartilage but rather a bulging of the airway membrane into the lumen during expiration.
- Bronchospasm is a mechanism of airway obstruction occurring when histamine is released from mast cells (in response to an allergy, irritant, or drug), causing a constriction of the muscular walls of the bronchioles.
- Mucosal inflammation and edema is fairly self-explanatory as a mechanism of airway obstruction; inflammatory cells accumulate in the mucosa (due to mucosal irritation), resulting in an increase in vascular permeability, and subsequent edema (swelling). This mechanism is seen in patients with COPD (a disease complex that includes chronic bronchitis and emphysema).
- Mucinous gland hypertrophy is a result of chronic stimulation of the glands (also seen in COPD); the glands increase in size, obstructing the airway lumen.
- External compression of the airway is also fairly self-explanatory; this is typically due to presence of a tumor pressing on the airway.

Endocrine

Diabetes Insipidus

Diabetes insipidus (DI) has a much different origin (origins, really) than that of the more well known diabetes mellitus (DM). Both DI and DM are characterized by an increase in urine production, which may be the most notable, and therefore the presenting, symptom. The urine collected from patients with DI, however, is strikingly different in that, in addition to the low specific gravity, it also has a low osmolality. The dilute urine eliminates DM from the differential. DI, rare as it is, has 4 possible causes. Nephrogenic DI occurs when the kidney's collecting tubules (where the urine is concentrated) become resistant to antidiuretic hormone (ADH). Primary polydipsia occurs when the patient drinks excessive amounts of water, diluting the concentration of ADH. Gestational DI is a result of increased ADH metabolism in pregnant women. The most common cause of DI, however, is trauma in which the pituitary is damaged.

Diabetes Mellitus

Complications of diabetes mellitus result in increased risk of multiple infections for the diabetic patient. Diabetic patients who suffer from diabetic neuropathy (or peripheral sensory neuropathy) are sometimes unaware of trauma to the distal extremities. Combined with the vascular insufficiency that is common in diabetic patients, poor wound healing ensues. This leaves the diabetic patient susceptible to infection, particularly anaerobic bacterial infections such as Clostridium perfringens, the causative agent of gangrene. Diabetic patients, especially those who do not have their disease under control, often suffer from Candida infections, due to the presence of glucose in the urine. Pseudomonas aeruginosa is a common cause of outer ear infections in diabetic patients. Sinus infection caused by saprophytic fungi (most commonly Rhizopus and Mucor) is also seen; this type of infection is called rhinocerebral mucormycosis.

Thyroid Storm

Thyroid storm (aka thyrotoxic crisis) occurs in hyperthyroid patients when the body is pushed past the threshold of being able to maintain metabolic function through compensation. This is a life-threatening state. Patients presenting with thyroid storm typically are hyperthermic, tachycardic, and in a state of anxiety or agitation. It is important to ask the patient whether he or she has any other existing conditions, and whether or not he or she has been sick lately; this is because thyroid storm is often triggered by acute illness. The defining lab value is a marked increase in free T4 (thyroxine) with a not so marked increase in total T4.

Addison Disease

Addison disease occurs when the adrenal cortex functions below baseline. The adrenal cortex is the rim of tissue that surrounds the bulk of adrenal tissue, the medulla. The cortex is responsible for the production of aldosterone, cortisol, and weak androgens. Dysfunction of the cortex can either result from a deficiency intrinsic to the gland (primary adrenal insufficiency) or from impaired secretion of adrenocorticotropic hormone (ACTH) by the pituitary gland (secondary adrenal insufficiency). Addison disease can result through a number of different mechanisms, including destruction of the adrenal cortex by antibodies (autoimmune adrenalitis, the most common cause of Addison), infection (AIDS, tuberculosis [TB]), or adrenal hemorrhage (Waterhouse-Friderichsen syndrome).

Neurologic

Glial Cells

There are 2 types of cells that comprise the central nervous system: neurons and glial cells. Glial cells function to support and protect neurons. There are 5 types of glial cells:

- Astrocytes: These cells are the link between neurons and vessels, controlling nutrient and electrolyte concentration. They also form part of the blood-brain barrier, which aids in keeping foreigners (e.g., bacteria, viruses) from traveling to the brain through the blood.
- Oligodendrocytes: These cells produce the myelin, which coats the axons of neurons to allow for conduction of impulses from neuron to neuron across synapses.
- Ependymal cells: These cells are responsible for the production and circulation of cerebrospinal fluid; they also form the lining of the brain's ventricles.
- Schwann cells: These cells perform the same functions as oligodendrocytes, only they are responsible for myelination of axons in the peripheral nervous system.
- Satellite cells: These cells protect neurons in the peripheral nervous system.

Transient Ischemic Attack

A transient ischemic attack (TIA) is defined as a temporary disruption of blood flow to the brain, causing neurologic effects that resolve within 24 hours. TIAs are sometimes referred to as "mini-strokes," and immediate treatment is necessary to prevent the development of stroke.

Stroke

A stroke is characterized by a rapid loss of neurologic function due to a disruption of cerebral blood flow. Symptoms of both stroke and TIA include paresthesia and hemiparesis, as well as loss of vision and aphasia (difficulty speaking); these symptoms are resolved quickly in the event of a TIA, but often remain permanently with stroke. A stroke can result either from ischemia (blockage of blood flow due to embolism or thrombosis) or hemorrhage (most commonly intercerebral or subarachnoid).

Brain Tumors

The most common type of primary brain tumor is glioblastoma multiforme (WHO grade IV astrocytoma). Meningioma, a benign tumor of the meningeal covering of the brain, is next, followed by low-grade astrocytoma (WHO grade II astrocytoma).

Individuals with a higher risk of developing a primary brain tumor include those with neurofibromatosis or tuberous sclerosis, as well as those with a family history of cancer. Patients with a brain tumor typically complain of headache, nausea, and vomiting, as well as a change in personality and progressive neurological deficits. For some patients, seizure is the first symptom of brain tumor. CT scan, MRI, and PET scan are all useful in diagnosing a brain tumor.

Renal/Genitourinary/Gynecologic

Proteinuria

Proteinuria, or protein in the urine (over 150 mg per 24 hours), has a variety of benign, self-limiting causes, including intense exercise, acute illness, dehydration, and fever. Prolonged proteinuria is a result of 1 of 3 pathophysiologic mechanisms: glomerular, tubular, or overflow proteinuria. Glomerular disease, which is the most common cause of pathologic proteinuria, is the result of increased permeability of the glomerular capillaries. These capillaries are fenestrated, meaning that they are intentionally "leaky"; this allows for glomerular filtration. These fenestrations are small enough to restrict the passage of larger protein molecules into the urine; in the diseased glomerulus, however, these large proteins are leaked through into the urine. In patients with tubular disease, the proximal convoluted tubule does not reabsorb low molecular weight proteins from the glomerular filtrate, causing these proteins to be excreted into the urine. Overflow proteinuria is the result of overproduction of certain proteins; this occurs in diseases such as multiple myeloma and other gammopathies.

Chronic Renal Failure

Glomerular filtration rate (GFR) and creatinine clearance are used to evaluate the severity of chronic renal failure. The serum creatinine level can be used to estimate the GFR because decreased glomerular filtration will always result in an increase in the serum creatinine; this can be used as a quick determination of glomerular function. For a more accurate picture of glomerular function, however, the GFR must be calculated. For men, GFR is calculated by subtracting the patient's age from 140. This number is then multiplied by the patient's weight in kilograms. This number is then divided by the patient's serum creatinine times 72. For women, the same formula is used only the final number is multiplied by 0.85. Another equally accurate method of determining GFR is calculating the creatinine clearance. Creatinine clearance is equal to the patient's urine creatinine times the 24-hour urine volume divided by serum creatinine times 1,440.

Hemodialysis

Patients with end-stage renal disease (ESRD) eventually require hemodialysis, typically when the creatinine clearance is less than 10 mL/min. Hemodialysis is an effective replacement for blood filtration in patients whose kidneys can no longer perform that duty. Even though the hemodialysis patient is carefully monitored before, during, and after dialysis treatments, more than a few complications exist. It is very important that a fluid balance is maintained at all times; many dialysis patients suffer from episodes of hypertension, when too much fluid is filtered and not enough is replaced. Muscle cramps are another common complication, occurring when the patient drinks too much fluid between treatments, necessitating removal of a larger volume of fluid in a short period of time. Not just fluid balance but electrolyte balance is important; an increase or decrease in serum potassium can cause arrhythmias and chest pain during dialysis as well. Circulation of blood through the dialysis machine invariably increases red cell hemolysis, which, over time, can lead to anemia in the dialysis patient.

Fournier Gangrene

Fournier gangrene is a relatively uncommon but serious necrotizing infection of the genital area; it is more common in men than women. Although uncommon among the general population, is not uncommon among patients with diabetes mellitus. It is also more commonly seen in immunosuppressed (patients with HIV, patients undergoing chemotherapy) patients, malnourished patients, and chronic alcoholic patients. The disease is caused typically by an infection of both aerobic and anaerobic organisms, and Clostridium perfringens is often identified. Because of the rapidly fatal progression of the infection, it is important to recognize the signs and begin treatment immediately. Fournier gangrene should be suspected when a red plaque is identified on the genitals; the plaque will quickly become purulent and necrotic-appearing; the tissue surrounding may be crepitant because of gas formation from the anaerobic bacteria.

Benign Prostatic Hyperplasia

Benign prostatic hyperplasia (BPH) is a common condition in middle-aged and elderly men. It is a noncancerous growth of the prostate caused by an increase in the number of prostatic stromal cells. The proliferation of these stromal cells results in the formation of discrete nodules in the prostate. The nodules are almost always located in the transition zone of the prostate (as opposed to most prostate cancers, which arise in the peripheral zone), which is the area surrounding the prostatic urethra. Due to the location of the nodules, the urethra becomes compressed as they grow, resulting in an increase in frequency of urination, as well as urinary urgency. The urethra may become blocked over time, resulting in bladder distension and infection. Alpha blockers and 5-alpha reductase inhibitors can provide relief from symptoms, but will not stop the progression of nodule growth. A surgical procedure called transurethral resection of the prostate (TURP) can provide relief because it removes the tissue that is compressing the urethra.

Polycystic Ovarian Syndrome

Polycystic ovarian syndrome (PCOS) is a disease of ovarian dysfunction that occurs when the ovaries are over stimulated by excess luteinizing hormone and insulin, which, in turn, causes the ovaries to produce an excess amount of androgens. Although the cause or causes of PCOS are as yet unclear, there is a strong association between PCOS and insulin resistance. Patients who are insulin resistant (but have no disorder of insulin production) have higher levels of insulin in the blood, which may cause over stimulation of the ovaries. However, not all insulin-resistant women develop PCOS, which suggests there may be some genetic component to the disease. In addition to insulin resistance, PCOS has been linked to frank diabetes mellitus, as well as obesity. Symptoms of PCOS include irregular menstruation or absent periods, infertility (due to anovulation), and depression. Symptoms that result from increased androgens include acne, male-pattern hair loss, and increased body and facial hair.

Gastrointestinal

Gastroesophageal Reflux Disease

Gastroesophageal reflux disease (GERD) has many contributing factors. Individuals with hiatal hernia (protrusion of the upper part of the stomach through the diaphragm) are thought to be at increased risk of developing GERD; gastroparesis (delayed emptying of the stomach) is also thought to play a role. The most significant cause of GERD, however, is a decrease in the muscle tone of the lower esophageal sphincter (LES), the muscular ring that controls the gastroesophageal junction. The LES, being composed of involuntary smooth muscle, is thus affected by hormones, drugs, and the body's own nervous system. Decreased LES tone is attributed to estrogen, progesterone, secretin, anticholinergics, and calcium channel blockers, as well as alcohol use, poor diet (high fat intake), and cigarette smoking. Complications include chronic esophagitis, Barrett esophagus (esophageal metaplasia), and esophageal adenocarcinoma.

Hepatitis

<u>Hepatitis A:</u>
This type of hepatitis is contracted through the fecal-oral route. Symptoms (nausea, vomiting, and fever) typically appear within 30 days of exposure to the virus. Hepatitis A is self-limiting, meaning that it will run its course and will not progress to the chronic stage of infection.

Hepatitis B:
This type of hepatitis is transmitted through the blood of an infected individual; though it may also be passed through body fluids that contain blood, including semen, saliva, vaginal fluid, and breast milk. Symptoms, if they appear, will typically present within 12 weeks of infection. Hepatitis B infection may be self-limiting, or it may transform into a chronic infection.

Hepatitis C:
This type of hepatitis is also passed through blood and body fluids that contain blood; symptoms (nausea, vomiting, fever, abdominal tenderness, jaundice, pruritus) present approximately 7 weeks after infection. About half of all patients infected with hepatitis C will progress to a chronic state.

Hepatitis D:
This type of hepatitis cannot infect on its own; it requires simultaneous infection with hepatitis B. The symptoms, progression, and outcome of hepatitis B/D coinfection are similar to infection with hepatitis B alone.

Hepatitis E:
Like hepatitis A, this type is also transmitted via the fecal-oral route, and has similar symptoms, though hepatitis E is more likely to progress to fulminant hepatitis.

Crohn Disease And Ulcerative Colitis

Crohn disease and ulcerative colitis (UC) are often confused with one another. However, there are striking differences between the two. Presentation for both diseases is variable, though diarrhea is very common for both, as is abdominal pain, cramping, and distention. Diarrhea associated with Crohn disease usually occurs a few times a week, usually after meals, and is not remarkable for blood or mucus. UC, on the other hand, is associated with multiple bouts of bloody diarrhea with mucus daily. UC is limited to the colon, while Crohn disease may present anywhere along the alimentary tract, though most cases involve the terminal ileum and cecum. Because only the colon is involved in UC, surgical removal of the colon is considered curative in patients with fulminant disease. Crohn disease, on the other hand, is not considered curative by surgery. The pattern of inflammation in UC is limited to the mucosa, while Crohn disease is more severe, often with transmural (involving the entire thickness of the wall) inflammation.

Hematology/oncology

Acute Myelogenous Leukemia

Acute myelogenous leukemia (AML) is a cancer of the myeloid stem cell line, and can occur anywhere along the maturation timeline for any of the cells from the myeloid progeny, including red blood cells, platelets, monocytes, and granulocytes. AML is most common in adults older than 65 years of age, although there is an incidence of the disease in the third decade of life, as well as in children younger than 2 years of age. Symptoms develop rapidly, and include fatigue, pallor, easy bruisability, petechial rash, shortness of breath, epistaxis, fever, and weight loss. The majority of these symptoms are attributed to bone marrow involvement of the disease, causing anemia and thrombocytopenia, which reflect in the labs as low hemoglobin, low hematocrit, and low platelet count. White blood cell count is high, and there is a marked hypercellularity in the bone marrow and the peripheral blood due to an increase in the production of immature white blood cells (or nucleated red blood cells or megakaryocytes, depending on the type of AML).

Melanoma

Although melanoma is less common than the other skin cancers (basal cell carcinoma and squamous cell carcinoma), it is responsible for the majority of skin cancer deaths. Melanoma is an invasive tumor that metastasizes very quickly; once the tumor has invaded past a certain depth or has spread to the lymphatics, the survival rate drastically decreases (estimated 5-year survival is less than 10%). Excision of the tumor before it spreads, however, is typically curative; thus early detection is extremely important. To help identify possible melanoma lesions, the mnemonic device ABCDE was developed. A stands for asymmetry of the lesion, B for irregular borders of the lesion, C for colors (melanomas may be irregularly colored, with multiple colors and shades), D for diameter (melanomas are usually greater than 5 mm), and E for elevation (melanomas are often raised lesions).

Ovarian Cancer

Although there are no direct causes that have been definitively linked to ovarian cancer, there are multiple factors that are attributed to the risk of developing the disease. Perhaps the strongest indicator that a woman may develop ovarian cancer is a genetic mutation of either the BRCA1 or BRCA2 gene, which also carries an increased risk of developing breast cancer. Increased age is associated with an increased risk of ovarian cancer, as is young age at menarche, and nulliparity. Conversely, multiparity and the use of oral contraceptives are linked to a reduced risk of developing ovarian cancer. Although ovarian cancer is notorious for its lack of symptoms (and thus its advanced stage at diagnosis), there are a few (however general) symptoms that are associated with ovarian cancer, including pelvic pain, bloating, urinary urgency, and feeling full very quickly when eating.

Immunology

Aids

Clinical category C: Clinical category C is for HIV-infected individuals who exhibit conditions that indicate that the patient has progressed to AIDS status; the HIV-positive patient will develop more opportunistic infections as his or her immune system becomes more compromised as a result of decreasing CD4 counts. Conditions that indicate that the patient has progressed to AIDS status include esophageal, tracheal, bronchial, or pulmonary candidiasis; cervical cancer; disseminated fungal infections, including coccidioidomycosis, histoplasmosis, and cryptococcosis; cytomegalovirus infection with widespread involvement; chronic herpes simplex infection; intestinal fungal infections, including cryptosporidiosis and isosporiasis; Kaposi sarcoma; lymphoma; disseminated Mycobacterium infection (tuberculosis, mycobacterium avium intracellulare, Mycobacterium kansasii); pneumocystic pneumonia and other recurrent pneumonias; CNS infections, including toxoplasmosis; HIV wasting syndrome.

Systemic Lupus Erythematosus

Systemic lupus erythematosus (SLE) is a chronic inflammatory disease of auto immunologic origin that involves multiple systems, targeting especially the skin, joints, and kidneys. It is more common in women than men, and has a peak incidence in the reproductive years. SLE can be a difficult disease to diagnose, because the initial symptoms are often vague and nonspecific. Mild to moderate anemia and an increased erythrocyte sedimentation rate are clues to the disease, but, again, these are nonspecific. Definitive diagnosis is made with a positive antinuclear antibody (ANA) test, along with a constellation of symptoms that include the following: malar rash (a red butterfly-shaped rash across the bridge of the nose and the cheeks); discoid rash (a raised scar-like lesion); photosensitivity; painful ulcers in the nose and mouth; nonspecific arthritis; pericarditis and/or pleuritis (serous inflammation of the pericardial sac and lining of the chest wall); proteinuria due to glomerular basement membrane damage; pancytopenia; antibodies to double-stranded DNA.

Musculoskeletal

Traumatic Fracture

In instances of traumatic fracture, the possibility of fat embolism should be considered; this is especially true in fractures involving the long bones (femur, humerus). When the bone is fractured, this allows for some of the fatty marrow contained within the bone to escape. Because the fracture and subsequent trauma to the area surrounding the fracture results in broken vessels, it is possible that the fatty marrow can be introduced into the bloodstream. When this happens, the events are similar to that of a deep venous thrombosis; the fat embolus dislodges from the lumen of the vessel and travels to the lung. When the embolus enters the pulmonary circulation, it eventually blocks blood flow as the caliber of the vessel through which it travels decreases, keeping blood from flowing to the lung tissue. The disruption in blood flow results in inflammation and necrosis of the lung, and eventually pulmonary failure ensues.

Degenerative Joint Disease

Degenerative joint disease (DJD), also known as osteoarthritis, is a disease of painful, inflamed joints. The pathological mechanism behind degenerative joint disease is twofold: one, the cartilage that acts as a cushion between bones becomes worn and thin, increasing the friction between the bones, and two, the amount of lubricating fluid inside the joint, called synovial fluid, is decreased, which exacerbates the friction. DJD is classified either as primary, meaning that it is related to the aging process, or secondary, meaning that there is another underlying cause of the disease. Secondary DJD may be caused by obesity, pregnancy, diabetes mellitus, previous injury to the joint, and storage disorders such as Wilson disease and hemochromatosis.

Common Problems in Acute Care

Fever

<u>Laboratory tests:</u>
When a patient has a fever, often the cause of the fever is not obvious. For this reason, laboratory tests, along with a thorough physical examination, can point the health care provider in the right direction. A white blood cell count should always be ordered. Although an elevated white cell count is not specific for infection, it is a positive indicator. Specifically, the presence of immature white cells in the blood (called a "left shift") is indicative of infection, because it means that white cells are being produced at an increased rate. A urinalysis should also be ordered to rule out a urinary tract infection as the cause of the fever, and a chest x-ray should be performed to rule out pneumonia. Blood cultures should also be ordered. If it is determined that the patient needs an antibiotic, a serum creatinine should be ordered to determine renal function because certain antibiotics should not be used in the setting of impaired renal function.

Shock

Hypovolemic shock:

Hypovolemic shock occurs when the volume of extracellular fluid (which is comprised of interstitial, intervascular, and transcellular fluids) is decreased to a significant degree (usually defined as a loss of at least one-fifth of the total blood volume); this type of shock can be due to severe loss of fluids (diarrhea and vomiting are common culprits, as well as profuse bleeding) or a decrease in fluid intake. Another less well-known cause of hypovolemia is a process called "third spacing," in which a large amount of fluid is moved into body cavities where it cannot be used; an example of this is the presence of ascites in the peritoneal cavity. Although the heart is functioning normally, the organs are not receiving an adequate supply of blood because of the decreased volume; the low blood volume results in low blood pressure (in severe cases, the blood pressure can be undetectable).

Multiple-organ failure syndrome:

The multiple-organ failure syndrome is defined as failure of 2 or more organ systems. The syndrome is recognized in patients who have been revived from the shock state, and occurs as a result of the body's natural systemic response to shock. Typically within 2 to 3 days of resuscitation, the systemic response is initiated; the degree of this response (largely inflammatory in nature) is dependent on the severity of the initial injury caused by the shock state. Although this inflammatory response typically resolves on its own within 2 weeks, in some patients a sustained elevated inflammation may be noted. The persistent inflammatory response results in a continued increase in cell production, which leads to a hypermetabolic, acidotic state, and this results in the progressive failure of the organs.

Nutritional imbalances

Syndrome of inappropriate secretion of ADH:

Syndrome of inappropriate secretion of ADH (SIADH) is defined as hyponatremia (a serum sodium level less than 135 mEq/L) with hypoosmolality (meaning that there is not an accompanying loss of water). A sodium level of less than 120 mEq/L is considered to be critical; seizure may result. Head trauma resulting in a severance of the pituitary stalk causes SIADH by disrupting the ADH feedback loop. Intracranial hemorrhage, encephalitis, and stroke may also cause SIADH. Extracranial causes of SIADH include lung oat cell carcinoma, lymphoma, thymoma, pancreatic adenocarcinoma, and lung infections (especially pneumonia and tuberculosis). Drugs known to cause SIADH include cyclophosphamide, chlorpropamide, carbamazepine, and nonsteroidal anti-inflammatory drugs (NSAIDs).

Acid-base imbalances

The four types of acid-base disturbances are respiratory acidosis, respiratory alkalosis, metabolic acidosis, and metabolic alkalosis. Respiratory acidosis occurs when the patient is in a state of hypoventilation; because the patient is not expiring carbon dioxide adequately on exhalation, the excess carbon dioxide accumulates in the blood, decreasing the pH. Respiratory alkalosis, on the other hand, occurs in the hyperventilative state; the blood pH increases because of increased loss of carbon dioxide. Metabolic acidosis results from either an increased loss of bicarbonate (through severe diarrhea, for example, which is commonly seen in children) or an increased production of acid (ketoacidosis). Metabolic alkalosis occurs when the level of bicarbonate in the blood is elevated; this can occur as a result of vomiting, or through excess ingestion of bicarbonate.

Drug toxicities

Assessing a patient with suspected drug overdose or toxin ingestion can be very difficult; time is of the essence in determining what was ingested so that the patient can be treated immediately. However, many of these patients are unresponsive and thus unable to communicate what exactly they ingested. Many drugs and toxins will leave clues, however, and some can be recognized by a specific odor. A sweet acetone smell is characteristic of multiple drugs and toxins, including grain alcohol, isopropyl alcohol, trichloroethane, chloroform, paraldehyde, and lacquer. An acetone odor is also strongly associated with patients in diabetic or alcoholic ketoacidosis. A garlic odor may be indicative of thallium, arsenic, selenium, or dimethyl sulfoxide toxicity. A violet smell is associated with turpentine ingestion, while cyanide has a characteristic almond odor, and zinc phosphide smells like raw fish.

Amphetamine:
The patient suffering from amphetamine toxicity will be hypertensive, hyperthermic, tachycardic, and tachypneic. Mental status may range from agitation to frank toxic psychosis, and the patient will appear hyperactive, hyperalert, and possibly paranoid. Clinical findings include dilated pupils (mydriasis), excessive sweating (diaphoresis), flushing, and hyperactive bowel sounds (borborygmi). Significant lab findings include elevated creatine phosphokinase.

Cocaine:
A cocaine overdose will present with hypertension, tachycardia, and hyperthermia, and the patient will appear agitated and anxious. Paranoia is more common in cocaine overdose, with some patients suffering from hallucinations. Clinical findings are similar to amphetamine overdose, with the addition of seizure and perforated nasal septum (accompanied by epistaxis). An elevated creatine phosphokinase is also seen in cocaine overdose, and electrocardiogram (ECG) abnormalities may be noted.

Opiate:
The patient suffering from an overdose of opioids will present in a hypotensive, hypothermic, bradycardic, bradypneic state. The mental status of an opioid

overdose patient can range from lethargy to coma, depending on the severity of the intoxication. The patient will move very slowly (if at all), and exhibit slurred speech. Pupils will be constricted (miosis), and bowel sounds will be diminished or absent. Arterial blood gas values will reflect respiratory acidosis, with an increase in blood carbon dioxide concentration.

Carbamazepine:
Carbamazepine is an anticonvulsant commonly used to treat epilepsy, though it is also used as a mood stabilizer in patients suffering from bipolar disorder. An overdose of carbamazepine will result in a hypotensive, tachycardic, bradypneic, hypothermic patient. The patient will appear lethargic, or may even be comatose. Oddly, an overdose of this drug may result in seizure, as well as hallucinations. The patient may have dilated pupils, and may also suffer from nystagmus. ECG abnormalities related to tachycardia are noted.

Wound management

Inflammatory phase of wound healing:
Immediately after tissue injury (within 5 to 10 minutes), epinephrine, norepinephrine, thromboxane, and prostaglandins are released; these mediators initiate vasoconstriction, which functions to control any hemorrhage in the area. This is followed by endothelial retraction, which exposes collagen on the subendothelium. Platelets attach to the collagen using fibrinogen, and the attached platelets then attract other platelets to form a platelet plug; this process is called platelet adhesion and aggregation. The aggregated platelets, which are now activated, release serotonin, histamine, and platelet-derived growth factor (PDGF) to initiate the coagulation cascade. The end result of the cascade is the activation of thrombin, which serves 2 purposes: to convert fibrinogen to fibrin, and to increase vascular permeability. The increase in permeability allows inflammatory cells to move from the bloodstream into the injured tissue. Neutrophils dominate the inflammatory picture in the early stages, and are later replaced by monocytes and tissue macrophages, which clean up the debris. Vasodilation increases the blood flow to the area to deliver more cells, fluid, and nutrients, and contributes to tissue edema.

Proliferative phase of wound healing:
The proliferative phase of wound healing begins at the end of the inflammatory phase (there is some overlap), usually within 3 to 5 days after the initial injury. Epithelialization is important; the purpose is to create a new layer of epithelium over the surface of the wound. In simple terms, this is a 2-step process: the epithelial cells proliferate from the edges of the wound and grow toward the center as the clot is dissolved. The epithelial cells secrete enzymes to stimulate the formation of plasmin, which slowly dissolves the clot as the epithelial layer is forming. Under the epithelial surface, fibroblasts are synthesizing and depositing collagen and elastin to restore the tissue to its pre-injured state. New blood vessels are formed during this

time (a process called angiogenesis) to deliver enzymes, macrophages, and other nutrients and cells. The blood vessels disappear as the need for them decreases. At the end of this phase, the wound tightens as the cells at the periphery contract.

Maturation phase of wound healing:
The maturation phase of wound healing consists mostly of the remodeling of collagen in the wound. Collagen remodeling is a somewhat complex process in which collagen is both removed and synthesized. The removal of old collagen from the wound occurs as a result of various enzymes, including collagenases and matrix metalloproteinases. During this remodeling process, type III collagen is slowly replaced by type I collagen, and proteoglycans replace hyaluronic acid, while water is reabsorbed from the area. This eliminates spaces between collagen fibers, and promotes a more orderly distribution of fibers, thus reducing the size of the scar over time.

Nosocomial infections

A nosocomial infection is an infection that a patient develops during his or her hospital stay; it also may be called a hospital-acquired infection, or a health care–associated infection. For an infection to be considered nosocomial, it must occur 48 hours or more after the patient is admitted to the hospital, to be sure that the patient was not infected prior to admission. An infection may also be considered nosocomial if it develops within 30 days of the patient's discharge from the hospital. Some infections, when introduced to a patient, can spread like wildfire from one patient to another if proper precautions are not taken.

Transmission:
There are 6 known routes of microorganism transmission involved in the spread of infection. The first mode is direct-contact transmission, in which an organism is transferred from an infected individual to a susceptible individual through direct bodily contact. Indirect-contact transmission occurs when an infected individual touches and contaminates an object (phone, sink, glove), and the object transmits the organism to another individual. Common vehicle transmission is similar to indirect-contact transmission, but the organism is transmitted through food, water, or medication. When an infected individual coughs or sneezes, organism-containing droplets can land on another individual, resulting in droplet transmission. Airborne transmission is similar, except that the organisms within the droplets can remain suspended in the air for long periods of time and be inhaled by another individual. A less common mode of transmission in hospitals is vector-borne transmission, in which organisms are transferred to the individual through a carrier such as a mosquito.

Common nosocomial offenders:
Any patient in the hospital can acquire a nosocomial infection, although children, burn victims, post-surgical patients, and the immunocompromised (e.g., oncology

patients, HIV-infected patients, post-transplant patients) are at much greater risk. Common bacterial nosocomial infections are caused by Escherichia coli, Proteus mirabilis, Pseudomonas aeruginosa, Klebsiella pneumoniae, Clostridium difficile, Acinetobacter species, and Citrobacter species (all of which are gram-negative), as well as Streptococcus pneumoniae and Staphylococcus aureus (both of which are gram-positive). Fungal agents may also cause nosocomial infection, especially the yeasts Candida albicans and Candida glabrata. Common viral causes of nosocomial infection include respiratory syncytial virus (RSV), rhinovirus, influenza, parainfluenza, and enteroviruses.

Precautions:
Perhaps the most important guidelines for the prevention of transmission between both patients and health care workers are the Universal Precautions guidelines, which state that every patient should be regarded as potentially infectious with regard to handling anything that could potentially transmit a blood-borne pathogen (such as the HIV virus or hepatitis C virus). This includes the handling of blood, tissue, semen, vaginal secretions, and body cavity fluids (synovial, cerebrospinal, pleural, pericardial, peritoneal, and amniotic). Treating every patient as potentially infectious ensures that the most care is taken to protect all patients. This includes wearing gloves (and changing them between patients), gowns, and other protection as necessary. Disposable items should be used whenever possible, and items that cannot be discarded must be disinfected. Frequent and proper hand washing is also extremely important, and all health care workers should keep nails short and clean, as bacteria can hide under long nails and be transferred to patients.

Psychopathology

Referral to mental health specialists

An acute care nurse is trained to recognize psychological needs in his or her patient, and is often able to provide adequate care for the patient while he or she is a patient on the ward. However, there are certain situations that require the intervention of a mental health specialist, such as a psychiatrist. For example, if the patient is suffering from a complex illness or constellation of illnesses, it may be difficult to evaluate his or her psychological health. If the patient has been receiving treatment, and improvements are not seen, a consultation may also be required. Patients with both mental health issues and substance abuse problems require evaluation and treatment by a mental health specialist, as do patients with illnesses that require behavioral therapy. If the acute care nurse feels that the patient is at a high risk for committing suicide, further psychiatric care must be provided.

Depression

Like anxiety, depression can be strictly a psychiatric diagnosis, or it may be the result of an underlying medical condition. Individuals suffering from depression are sometimes written off by their physicians and nurses without further investigation as to the actual cause; it is important that the doctor or nurse really listen to the patient and try to determine the origin of the depression because an underlying cause must be identified. Diseases and conditions that are linked to depression include diabetes, hypothyroidism, Addison disease (adrenal insufficiency), Cushing disease, AIDS, chronic fatigue syndrome, fibromyalgia, infectious mononucleosis, systemic lupus erythematosus, narcolepsy, multiple sclerosis, brain tumor, migraines, and sleep apnea.

Major depressive disorder:

An individual suffering from major depressive disorder will present with notably depressed mood, lethargy, and fatigue. He or she may complain of loss of appetite, as well as problems sleeping, which may vary from insomnia to hypersomnia, depending on the individual. Agitation and problems with concentration or the feeling of being in a "mental fog" are common, as well as lack of motivation and lack of interest in activities that once were found to be pleasurable/enjoyable. The patient with major depressive disorder may have a pervasive feeling of worthlessness, and may contemplate suicide. The diagnostic criteria for major depressive disorder include at least 1 month of depression without episodes of mania. Treatment includes selective serotonin reuptake inhibitors (SSRIs), mood stabilizers such as lithium and divalproex sodium, and psychotherapy. For patients with refractory depression, ECT may be an option.

Clinical features:

- Major depressive episode: characterized by sadness, loneliness, guilt, anxiety, irritability, anger, lethargy, apathy, inability to concentrate, insomnia or hypersomnia, loss of appetite, anhedonia, loss of libido, feelings of worthlessness, and suicidal ideation.
- Manic episode: characterized by an increase in energy, insomnia, short attention span, racing thoughts, impulsive behavior (spending sprees, drug/alcohol binges, and promiscuity), irritability, euphoria, and delusions of grandeur.
- Hypomanic episode: characterized by increased energy, creative thinking, racing thoughts, and uncontrollable laughter. Symptoms are usually not as severe as mania, and episodes are typically shorter.
- Mixed affective episode: characterized by symptoms of both mania and depression simultaneously, causing paranoia, confusion, anxiety or panic, fatigue, restlessness, insomnia, and suicidal ideation.

Substance abuse

Serotonin syndrome:

The serotonin syndrome is a state of serotonin toxicity caused either by overdose or drug interaction. The syndrome is the result of an increase in the level of serotonin in the central nervous system, and can be fatal if it is not recognized and treated immediately. There are 3 phases associated with the serotonin syndrome, and each phase has its own set of characteristic symptoms. A patient in the early phase of the serotonin syndrome is agitated, confused, restless, and diaphoretic, and may suffer from nausea, vomiting, diarrhea, myoclonic jerking, tremors, and flushing. Hypertension, hypertonicity, hyperthermia, and advanced myoclonus indicate that the patient is in the middle phase of the syndrome. In the late phase of toxicosis, the patient becomes acidotic, followed by respiratory and renal failure, disseminated intravascular coagulation (DIC), and rhabdomyolysis.

Blood alcohol concentration:
When an individual has consumed 1 or 2 drinks, his or her blood alcohol concentration is near 0.05%; although the individual may not be visibly intoxicated at this point, his or her judgment is impaired, however slightly. Ingestion of 5 or 6 alcoholic beverages (a blood alcohol concentration of about 0.1%) results in slowed response time and reflexes, and the individual may exhibit slurred speech and clumsiness. At a rate of 10 to 12 drinks, the blood alcohol concentration doubles, and the individual noticeably staggers or even has difficulty walking or standing; he or she may become unintelligible. The individual also exhibits extreme emotional responses, ranging from anger to tearfulness. At 15 to 18 drinks, the individual appears confused, and may be unresponsive (in a stupor). At blood alcohol levels above 0.4%, coma, respiratory depression, cardiac arrhythmias, and death can result. Remember, however, that everyone is different, and some individuals can tolerate alcohol better than others.

Alcohol withdrawal:
The symptoms of alcohol withdrawal range from mild to severe, and which symptoms the patient will experience depends upon how long they have been drinking as well as how much they drink on a regular basis. It is important to be able to recognize these symptoms and get an accurate history from the patient or the patient's family. Mild to moderate symptoms of withdrawal include headache, nausea, tachycardia, an increase in blood pressure, sweating, shaking, vomiting, and loss of appetite. For the chronic, severe alcoholic, more serious symptoms can occur with withdrawal, and the patient should be under medical care. These symptoms include delirium tremens (characterized by disorientation, confusion, hallucinations, hyperthermia, hypertension, and tachycardia), seizure, heart attack, and stroke.

Treatment: For the relief of mild to moderate withdrawal symptoms, benzodiazepines (particularly diazepam) are commonly used. These drugs have a calming effect on the central nervous system, and may help prevent seizure and delirium tremens. Benzodiazepines should be used for as short a time as possible to prevent the patient from becoming dependent and having to suffer through benzodiazepine withdrawal. Carbamazepine (an anti-seizure medication) may be used in place of a benzodiazepine. Beta-blockers are sometimes administered to control blood pressure and heart rate. Anti-seizure medications and lidocaine are used to help treat delirium tremens and seizure, while antipsychotics (such as haloperidol) are used for patients who are combative, aggressive, and/or psychotic.

Anxiety

Although anxiety can be strictly psychiatric in nature, there are various diseases and medical conditions that are known to cause some level of anxiety in afflicted individuals. In the case of certain illnesses, the anxiety may either be caused by the disease, or the anxiety may cause or exacerbate the disease. Anxiety is often associated with tachycardia of both ventricular and supraventricular origin, as well as other cardiovascular conditions, including myocardial infarction, congestive heart failure, and mitral valve prolapse. Endocrine diseases are also commonly related to anxiety, especially hyperthyroidism, hyperparathyroidism, and carcinoid syndrome. Irritable bowel syndrome is closely linked to anxiety, as is peptic ulcer disease. Neurological conditions associated with anxiety include epilepsy and other seizure disorders, Parkinson disease, and essential tremor.

Obsessive-compulsive disorder:
Obsessive-compulsive disorder (OCD) is an anxiety disorder in which the sufferer is overcome by obsessive thoughts and attempts to cancel out or neutralize those thoughts through the performance of compulsive rituals. To be classified as obsessive, the individual must have recurrent, pervasive, intrusive thoughts or impulses that cause anxiety for the individual; these thoughts are not related to real-life problems; the individual tries to suppress the thoughts or replace them with other thoughts or actions; and the individual is aware that the thoughts are a product of his or her mind. A compulsion is a repetitive act that the individual feels compelled to perform in order to neutralize an obsession, with the goal of reducing anxiety associated with that obsession. These compulsions continually disrupt the individual's daily activities.

Mood disorders

Although many people, health care providers included, are under the assumption that bipolar disorder is a single entity, in actuality it represents a spectrum of mood disorders. The disorders that fall along this spectrum are bipolar I, bipolar II, cyclothymia, and bipolar NOS (not otherwise specified). The diagnosis of bipolar I disorder is made when the patient experiences at least 1 episode of mania; the patient may also experience 1 or more depressive episodes, but these are not required for the diagnosis of bipolar I. The individual with bipolar II disorder experiences episodes of hypomania with 1 or more episodes of major depression. Cyclothymia is characterized by episodes of hypomania that alternate with episodes of depression; these depressive episodes do not meet the diagnostic criteria for major depression. Bipolar NOS is a diagnosis that is used for individuals who do not meet the criteria for any of the other bipolar disorders.

Diagnostic reasoning

Data Gathering

The gathering and recording of data are of utmost importance to the diagnostic evaluation process. The history and physical section of the patient chart contains a wealth of information (ideally), and should always be taken into consideration when developing a care plan for the patient. Because any number of clinicians can add information to the patient chart (and because all of these clinicians will be reading this information), it is important to record all information clearly and in an organized manner. This can be a daunting task when you consider all of the different sources of information, including the patient interview, family member interviews, previous charts, and lab results. By keeping this information clear and concise, you can minimize error, and you can be sure that the differential diagnosis is comprehensive.

Problems in data evaluation:
The data that are available on the patient chart are an integral part of the patient's overall care plan. However, errors may be present in the records, and these errors may negatively influence clinical decision making; thus it is important to look at the information as a whole. Does it make sense? Make sure that the patient's verbal history agrees with what you see in his or her records. Also, remember that not every test result you see in the patient's chart is necessarily accurate. If a test result doesn't make sense in the clinical picture as a whole, consider why this might be. It could simply be an error (e.g., the wrong number was recorded, the blood was drawn incorrectly), or the patient may have a result that would be considered "abnormal," though for this particular patient it is not. For example, a marathon runner may have a resting heart rate of 40 bpm; while this is a bradycardic rate, it is not pathological, but rather a result of physical conditioning.

Diagnostic testing

Sensitivity and specificity:
Some degree of error is inherent in almost all diagnostic testing. When you order a diagnostic test for a patient, how confident should you be that the result will be accurate? The terms sensitivity and specificity are used to illustrate the accuracy of diagnostic tests. The sensitivity of a test refers to its ability to correctly identify patients who do have the disease. If a test is administered to 100 patients with diabetes, and all 100 patients test positive, the test is considered to have a sensitivity of 100%. If only 85 of those tested have a positive result, however, that means that the test has a false-negative rate of 15%, and a sensitivity of 85%. On the other hand, the specificity of a diagnostic test refers to its ability to identify patients who do not have the disease. If 100 nondiabetic patients are tested for diabetes, and 50 of them have a positive result, the test has a specificity of only 50%.

Positive and negative predictive values:
Predictive values are of importance to the clinician because although sensitivity and specificity are used to evaluate the effectiveness of a diagnostic test, they are not particularly clinically relevant. Since a patient's disease state is more or less unknown at admission, these parameters are of no help. This is where the positive predictive value (PPV) and negative predictive value (NPV) of a test come in. If your patient tests positive for syphilis, what are the chances that the patient actually has syphilis? The chance that this result is correct is the PPV; this is calculated by dividing the number of true positive results by the number of total positive results (true and false positives). NPV, then, is the probability that a patient with a negative result really does not have syphilis. Dividing the number of true negatives by the number of total negatives will give you the NPV.

Universal principles of diagnostic testing:
First, it is important to remember that the positive and negative predictive values of a test are not absolute. For example, if you test a high-risk population for diabetes (say 180 out of 200 have the disease), and then you test a low-risk population (20 out of 200 have the disease), the sensitivity and specificity of the test will stay the same, but the predictive values will change. Also, a test that has less than 100% sensitivity and specificity is most useful for the patient with an equivocal or intermediate probability of disease, rather than a high-risk patient or a low-risk patient. One other important point to remember is that sensitivity and specificity are inversely related. If a diagnostic test is modified in order to increase its sensitivity, the specificity of the test will decrease, and vice versa.

Differential diagnosis

The differential diagnosis is an important tool that allows the clinician to familiarize him or herself with the patient's condition, understand the condition, create an effective treatment plan, and follow the progress of the patient. To start, thoroughly examine the patient's chart, making a list of all of the abnormal test results and laboratory values. Add to this list all of the patient's complaints. Once this list is complete, organize the test results, labs, and complaints by anatomic location or organ system. After breaking the list down by organ site, look for any relationships between symptoms and/or results. Create another list of those data that seem to be related, and list all of the diseases or conditions that explain the findings, eliminating any that do not fit.

Evidence-based medicine

Evidence-based medicine (EBM) is defined as the "conscientious, explicit, and judicious use of current best evidence in making decisions about the care of individual patients." The goal of the practice of evidence-based medicine is to take information gained from scientific study and apply it to the practice of medicine. In other words, the direct outcome of the study is used to assess practicality and efficacy in clinical practice. The goal of the studies behind EBM is to determine and identify all the risks associated with a particular treatment, as well as all the benefits. Once the risks and the benefits have been identified, they can be weighed against one another to determine the overall risk/benefit ratio for that particular treatment plan.

Physical Assessment

Patient history

The patient interview is the first step in the process of treating a patient, and it is often where the most important information is obtained. Because it is such a crucial part of the overall assessment of the patient, it is important to make the patient feel comfortable. You are not likely to get a great deal of information from a patient if you make a negative impression. If possible, conduct the interview in a quiet area. If this is not a possibility, remain calm and relaxed as you interview the patient, and take your time both when asking questions and listening to the answers. If you give the patient the impression that you are impatient or in a rush, he or she may become uncomfortable and hesitant to answer questions.

Obtaining accurate information:
Remember, the main goal of the interview is to get the most information you can, and to make sure that the information is accurate. Asking the patient open-ended questions allows for them to elaborate on their symptoms. Only ask one question at a time, so that the patient knows what question to respond to. Be sure to ask questions clearly, and do not use medical terms that could confuse the patient. After you have finished your questioning, you can repeat your notes back to the patient to make sure that you have accurately understood and recorded their complaints. If the patient has anything to add to the account, record that information as well.

Components of the patient history:
A comprehensive patient history contains numerous components to help the clinician formulate a diagnosis and treatment plan. Demographic information is an important part of the history, and includes information about the patient's age, sex, and race. The source of the patient referral is also included in the history; it is important to know whether the patient was referred by a primary care physician, a cardiologist, or some other doctor. If someone other than the patient is providing the history, his or her name should be recorded. The chief complaint, or the reason that the patient is being seen, is also important to note, along with a detailed history of the complaint, including when the patient first noticed symptoms, if the symptoms are better or worse at certain times, and what the characteristics of the illness are. Any past medical problems and surgeries are documented as well, including diseases and surgical procedures within the patient's family. Allergies, current medications, and social factors/practices are included in the history.

Screening tests: When the clinician is asking the patient about his or her past medical history, it is important that the clinician includes questions regarding screening tests that the patient may or may not have had recently. If the patient has not had appropriate screening, the clinician should investigate and consider ordering any tests that relate to the patient's current condition. Screening tests such as cholesterol, hemoglobin, and serum glucose are routine blood tests and can be done easily. Urinalysis is another simple screening test, as is a blood pressure reading. More involved and time-consuming tests can be ordered for patients when indicated, including sigmoidoscopy and stool guaiac for routine colon cancer screening, Papanicolaou smear for cervical dysplasia and cancer, mammogram for breast cancer, and ECG for heart abnormalities.

Clinical Management

National Standards of Practice

ANA and AACN

Mission:
The American Association of Critical-Care Nurses (AACN) provides and inspires leadership to establish work and care environments that are respectful, healing, and humane. The AACN's key to success is through its members. Therefore, the AACN is committed to providing the highest quality resources to maximize nurses' contribution to caring for critically ill patients and their families.

Vision:
The AACN is dedicated to creating a health care system driven by the needs of patients and families where critical care professionals make their optimal contribution.

Values:
In addition to its mission and vision, the AACN has also published a set of values intended for all AACN members to uphold. These values state that the AACN member will:

1. Be accountable for basing his or her practice on ethical actions and principles.
2. Advocate changes in the AACN organization that benefit patients and their families.
3. Practice with integrity, including honest communication, loyalty, and the honoring of promises and commitments.
4. Communicate and cultivate relationships with other AACN members.
5. Assume a leadership role, promoting strategic thinking, planning, and problem solving.
6. Meet and/or exceed all standards and expectations.
7. Remain a fair, impartial, and responsible leader.
8. Continue to make contributions through learning, questioning, and critical thinking.
9. Promote innovative thinking.
10. Remain committed and passionate about the organization, and inspire others to do the same.

Standards of care:

The American Nurses Association (ANA) and the American Association of Critical Care Nurses (AACN) have collaborated to provide published standards of care for the ACNP.

- Standard I states that the ACNP is responsible for collecting patient data.
- Standard II states that the ACNP is responsible for determining diagnoses by analyzing said data.
- Standard III states that the ACNP is responsible for identifying expected outcomes specific to the patient.
- Standard IV states that the ACNP is responsible for developing a care plan with specific interventions.
- Standard V states that the ACNP is responsible for implementing patient interventions.
- Standard VI states that the ACNP is responsible for evaluating the progress of the patient.

Standards of professional performance:

The ANA and the AACN collaborated to publish a set of standards of professional performance for the ANCP as follows:

- Standard I states that the ACNP will systematically evaluate the quality and effectiveness of acute care nursing as a practice.
- Standard II states that the ACNP will use available organizational resources (e.g., publications, conferences) to aid in patient care.
- Standard III states that the ACNP will use professional practice standards to evaluate his or her own practice.
- Standard IV states that the ACNP will maintain current acute care knowledge.
- Standard V states that the ACNP will contribute to the professional development of colleagues.
- Standard VI states that the ACNP will make ethical decisions and act accordingly.
- Standard VII states that the ACNP will form collaborations in providing patient care.
- Standard VIII states that the ACNP will use research findings in his or her practice.
- Standard IX states that the ACNP will deliver patient care safely and effectively.

High-acuity patients:

The acute care nurse practitioner will encounter more high-acuity patients than the nurse practitioner that works in, say, a family medicine clinic. High-acuity patients are patients whose conditions are more critical, less stable, and require more attention; emergency departments, operating rooms, and intensive care units are areas of the hospital that see a high volume of high-acuity patients. The ANA and the AACN have established a set of components that comprise the role of the acute care nurse practitioner when working with high-acuity patients. The ACNP should include the following components in the workup of every high-acuity patient: a comprehensive health history, a comprehensive physical examination, a health risk profile and analysis, a differential diagnosis based on diagnostic reasoning, a therapeutic intervention plan, and consultation with health care providers in other specialties.

ACNP's Scope of Practice

The ACNP's Scope of Practice identifies a number of areas in which the ACNP should be competent. The ACNP is expected to have an extensive working knowledge base, and he or she is also expected to have excellent communication skills. The ability to perform both a patient health history and a physical examination are central to the ACNP's scope of practice, as is the ability to both order and interpret laboratory tests and diagnostic procedures. In addition, the ACNP is expected to be able to perform certain invasive procedures, such as intensive wound care, to remove drains and staples, and to assist in surgical procedures. The ACNP is required to prescribe drugs, and monitor the effects of those drugs during the course of treatment. The ACNP must be organized, enthusiastic, intuitive, inventive, and respectful towards patients, families, and other health care professionals.

Pharmacotherapeutics

Cardiovascular pharmacotherapeutics

There are 10 different classes of drugs that are used to treat cardiovascular disease. Antianginal drugs are used to treat pain associated with hypoxic tissue (angina) by increasing the perfusion of the myocardium. Antiarrhythmic drugs treat cardiac arrhythmias by normalizing sinus rhythm. Antihypertensives and cardioinhibitory drugs reduce blood pressure; cardiostimulatory drugs increase heart rate and blood pressure. Diuretics promote urine production, reducing the blood volume, and thus reducing blood pressure. Pressors increase heart rate, cardiac output, and blood pressure. Vasoconstrictors increase venous blood pressure, while vasodilators decrease venous blood pressure. Thrombolytics are used to dissolve blood clots and thrombotic emboli.

<u>Atropine:</u>
Atropine is a drug known as a muscarinic receptor antagonist; the drug works by binding to muscarinic receptors, thus blocking acetylcholine from binding to the muscarinic receptors. Acetylcholine, when bound to muscarinic receptors, is responsible for increasing vagal stimulation of the heart; increased vagal stimulation of the heart, in turn, is responsible for slowing the heart rate. In patients with bradycardia resulting from an atrioventricular (AV) nodal block, atropine may be administered to correct the block. When atropine is administered to patients with an AV block, the drug binds to the muscarinic receptors, blocking the

acetylcholine from binding; this results in a decrease in vagal stimulation of the heart, which increases the heart rate.

Antihypertensives:

Primary (or essential) hypertension is responsible for approximately 95% of all cases of hypertension. It is called primary hypertension because it is not resultant of another disease process (as secondary hypertension is); in fact, the exact cause of primary hypertension is largely unknown. It has been linked to increases in both blood volume and cardiac output, and the response to treatment seems to support this theory. The class of drugs used to treat hypertension (called antihypertensives) generally operates under 1 or a combination of 3 mechanisms: reduction of systemic vascular resistance, reduction of blood volume, and reduction of cardiac output.

Pulmonary hypertension: Pulmonary arterial hypertension (PAH) is, in many cases, secondary to another illness or disease process. In these cases, the hypertension can usually be controlled by treating the underlying cause. In cases in which the cause of the hypertension is unknown (primary PAH), however, pharmacologic intervention may be effective. This can be a multi-pronged approach, as sometimes the use of multiple drugs results in better results. A vasodilator is used to decrease vascular resistance, lowering the arterial pressure. Most vasodilators are not specific for arteries, and thus relax and dilate veins as well. A drug called hydralazine, however, is specific for arterial dilation, and works well for PAH. Other drugs that may be used in concert with a vasodilator include a diuretic (to decrease blood volume), and anticoagulants (such as heparin) to prevent clot formation.

Tissue plasminogen activator:

Tissue plasminogen activator (tPA) is a thrombolytic agent used to dissolve blood clots before they cause irreversible damage to the heart, brain, or other organs. A blot clot is composed of red blood cells, white blood cells, platelets, and fibrin, among other things; when tPA is administered, it binds to the fibrin in the clot. The binding of tPA to fibrin activates another fibrin-bound protein called plasminogen; plasminogen, in its active form, is called plasmin. Plasmin is a strong enzymatic protease that plays a major role in clot lysis; when it is released from its fibrin-binding sites through the binding of tPA, it then breaks apart the fibrin molecules within the clot, initiating the clot-dissolving process.

Pulmonary pharmacotherapeutics

Theophylline:

Theophylline is an aromatic organic compound called dimethylxanthine, belonging to a group of methylxanthines. The mode of action of the drug is as a broad adenosine receptor antagonist; because it is not specific for a particular adenosine receptor, many of its effects are not intended. Theophylline is used mainly for the treatment of asthma and COPD, and it is very effective at treating these diseases. However, because of its nonspecificity, its levels must be monitored in all patients taking the drug to avoid toxicity. Theophylline works by relaxing the smooth muscle surrounding the bronchioles; increasing the heart rate, heart contractility, and blood pressure; increasing blood flow to the kidneys; and stimulating the respiratory center, which is located in the brainstem.

Tuberculosis:

Currently, the Centers for Disease Control and Prevention (CDC) recommends a 4-drug regimen for the treatment of tuberculosis. These 4 drugs are isoniazid, rifampin, pyrazinamide, and ethambutol. The regimen calls for the 4 drugs to be taken together for 8 weeks; pyrazinamide and ethambutol are then discontinued while the patient continues to take isoniazid and rifampin for the remaining 4 months. Two major problems exist regarding this treatment regimen: patient compliance and drug resistance. Patient noncompliance is common because of the nature of the side effects of the drugs. Most of these drugs, rifampin especially, have side effects that are not well tolerated by the patient. Isoniazid, rifampin, and pyrazinamide are each known to cause hepatitis; when the 3 are taken together, the risk of hepatitis increases, as do the side effects associated with hepatotoxicity. The other major problem associated with tuberculosis treatment is drug resistance; typically, drug regimens for tuberculosis only work for a period of time before the disease becomes resistant to the drugs.

Interstitial lung disease:

Interstitial lung disease (ILD) is actually a group of diseases characterized by a thickening of the alveoli and the tissue surrounding the alveoli (the interstitium). The thickening of the lung tissue is caused by inflammation and subsequent scarring and fibrosis; in some cases, the cause is known (e.g., sarcoidosis, asbestosis) and in others it is not (so-called idiopathic pulmonary fibrosis). ILD is a progressive disease; there is no absolute cure for the disease. Patients are treated with corticosteroids, which reduce the inflammation and swelling (due to the accumulation of fluid, or edema) of the interstitium. Immunosuppressive drugs may also be beneficial by helping to quell the inflammatory response. Drugs known as angiofibrotics are used to treat patients with ILD as well; these drugs can help slow the process of fibrosis, though they cannot reverse the damage that has already occurred. Patients with severe alveolar noncompliance and subsequent hypoxemia may require oxygen therapy, though this leads to further lung damage over time.

Endocrine pharmacotherapeutics

Artificial insulin:

Patients with type I diabetes mellitus are born with a defect in insulin production; these patients, then, rely on insulin injections to control their blood glucose levels because they do not produce the insulin necessary to regulate their blood glucose. There are several different kinds of insulin that may be used to control type I DM, and they are classified based on their speed of action. Rapid-acting insulin starts to work within approximately 10 minutes of injection, and the effects continue for 3 to

4 hours; this type of insulin is particularly effective for the patient in diabetic shock (ketoacidosis). Short-acting insulin takes a little longer to begin working, within 30 minutes, and lasts for 5 to 8 hours. Intermediate-acting begins working in 1 to 3 hours and lasts for approximately 16 to 24 hours; long-acting insulin begins working within 4 to 6 hours, and is active for 24 to 48 hours.

Vasopressin:

Vasopressin, or antidiuretic hormone (ADH), is used in a variety of clinical situations. The synthetic form of vasopressin, called desmopressin, is administered to patients either intravenously, nasally, or orally (in pill form). Desmopressin is most commonly used in the treatment of diabetes insipidus, a disease in which the kidney, because of a lack of vasopressin production, does not concentrate urine at the distal convoluted tubule. This results in frequent, excessive voiding of hypotonic urine. Patients with a decrease in vasopressin production benefit from desmopressin therapy. Desmopressin is also used to treat chronic bedwetting in children, and has been shown to improve clotting in individuals suffering from von Willebrand disease, thrombocytopenia, and mild cases of factor VIII deficiency (hemophilia A).

Hyperthyroidism:

Hyperthyroidism is a disease in which the thyroid tissue becomes overfunctional, producing large amounts of triiodothyronine and thyroxine (T3 and T4, respectively); this results in an excess of both of these hormones in the circulation. There are 2 groups of medications that are typically indicated in patients with hyperthyroidism; these medications do not cure the disease, but only control it, and they may lose effectiveness over time. Thyrostatic drugs, such as propylthiouracil, are used to prevent the conversion of thyroxine (which is mostly inactive) into triiodothyronine (the active thyroid hormone). Beta-blockers are also used in conjunction with thyrostatic drugs, though they are used for their palliative effects. An excess of circulating thyroid hormone causes stimulation of the sympathetic nervous system, resulting in anxiety, tremor, and increased heart rate; beta-blockers help to control these symptoms. For patients with disease that is refractory to thyrostatic treatment, radioiodine ablation therapy and surgical removal of the thyroid gland remain as viable treatment options.

Addison disease:

Addison disease, or adrenal insufficiency, is a result of underproduction of steroid hormones by the adrenal cortex. The adrenal cortex is responsible for the production of mineralocorticoids, glucocorticoids, and weak androgens; in Addison disease, there is a lack of these hormones. Maintenance therapy includes replacement of cortisol (a glucocorticoid that increases the blood glucose level in response to stress) with either hydrocortisone or prednisolone, as well as replacement of aldosterone (a mineralocorticoid responsible for the retention of sodium and water at the distal convoluted tubule) with fludrocortisone. An acute attack of Addison disease, called an Addisonian crisis, is a life-threatening medical emergency, and requires treatment with intravenous cortisone, saline, and glucose.

Neurologic pharmacotherapeutics

Levodopa:

Levodopa, or L-dopa, is a molecule that is the precursor to dopamine, epinephrine, and norepinephrine; it is widely used as a treatment for Parkinson's disease, a degenerative disease of the central nervous system that results in impaired production of dopamine. L-dopa is termed a "prodrug," which means that it is administered to the patient as an inactive drug; once L-dopa enters the body, it is then metabolized into dopamine, the active form, by dopa decarboxylase. The reason L-dopa is administered instead of the active dopamine is because the L-dopa molecule can cross the blood-brain barrier, whereas the dopamine molecule cannot; giving the patient dopamine, then, would be useless, because the dopamine would reside in the peripheral tissues instead of traveling to the brain, where it is needed. When L-dopa is administered, it crosses the blood-brain barrier into the brain, where it can then be metabolized into dopamine.

Problems: L-dopa, though it is the most effective drug (really, the only effective drug) for treatment of Parkinson disease, has a number of unpleasant side effects, including nausea, hair loss, anxiety, confusion, and visual hallucinations. The majority of these side effects can be attributed to the way that L-dopa is metabolized once it enters the body. The ideal situation would be that all of the L-dopa, once administered, would cross the blood-brain barrier into the brain, where it would be metabolized into dopamine. However, although the molecules can cross the barrier, not all of them do. The molecules that do not cross into the brain remain in the peripheral tissues, where they too are metabolized into dopamine. This peripheral dopamine supply causes a number of the adverse effects of the drug. To counteract this effect, a drug known as carbidopa, which prevents peripheral metabolization of L-dopa, is administered simultaneously.

Bacterial meningitis:

Bacterial meningitis is a very rapidly progressing infection of the membranous coverings of the brain (the meninges), and is highly fatal if untreated. In the United States, the most common causes of bacterial meningitis are Streptococcus pneumoniae and Neisseria meningitidis. S. pneumoniae, also called pneumococcus, requires a 2-week course of antibiotics; penicillin is the first line of defense for pneumococcus. For strains of pneumococcus that are resistant to penicillin, treatment is with ceftriaxone, cefotaxime, and/or vancomycin. N. meningitidis, or meningococcus, requires a week-long course of intravenous penicillin or ampicillin; for penicillin-resistant strains, ceftriaxone or cefotaxime is the treatment of choice. Listeria monocytogenes is a common cause of meningitis among neonates, and is treated with a 3-week course of intravenous gentamicin and ampicillin.

Haemophilus influenzae, a common cause among infants, is treated with either ceftriaxone or cefotaxime.

Status epilepticus:
Status epilepticus, a condition in which the sufferer is in a persistent state of seizure, has several causes, ranging from alcohol withdrawal to noncompliance in epileptic patients to brain tumor; some of these causes (e.g., brain tumor) do not respond to medication. For others, pharmacologic intervention may help control seizures. Benzodiazepines, especially diazepam and lorazepam, have proven to be very effective in controlling status epilepticus. Before the use of benzodiazepines, the most popular drugs for treating status epilepticus included barbiturates, such as sodium pentothal and pentobarbital, and phenytoin. Phenytoin and sodium pentothal are still used today for patients who are either refractory to or cannot tolerate treatment with benzodiazepines.

Renal, genitourinary, and gynecologic pharmacotherapeutics

Nephrotic syndrome:
Nephrotic syndrome is a group of diseases in which the renal capillaries are damaged by inflammation, causing them to become leaky; the damaged capillaries allow for protein and fluids to leak out into the surrounding tissue, causing edema. The causes of nephrotic syndrome are classified as either primary (those that are intrinsic to the kidney, though the exact cause is unknown) or secondary (those that result from other disease processes, such as lupus or diabetes). There is no cure for nephrotic syndrome, and the treatment depends on the cause. For the primary nephrotic syndromes, a diuretic such as furosemide is used to control fluid retention; maintenance of the disease includes monitoring of fluid intake and kidney function. For the secondary nephrotic syndromes, treatment is tailored to the underlying disease; for example, cyclosporin may be used to control autoimmune nephron damage, while diet may help reduce diabetic nephropathy.

Renal calculi:
There are many different types of renal calculi (kidney stones), and there are different risk factors and diseases associated with each. For the most part, however, diet modification is a good way to minimize the risk of kidney stone formation. Stones form in the kidney when certain minerals are present in high concentrations in the blood; dehydration contributes to the risk by further concentrating the minerals. Proper hydration is one of the best ways to prevent stone formation; drinking at least 2 liters of water a day will essentially “flush out” any debris that is present in the kidneys. Consuming foods that are low in sodium, nitrogen, and oxalate will reduce the risk of developing stones; patients who have suffered from stones in the past and are especially prone to them may also be placed on a low-protein diet. For patients with a predisposition to calcium stone formation, allopurinol may be an effective treatment as well.

Benign prostatic hyperplasia:

Benign prostatic hyperplasia (BPH) is a common problem in men older than 50 years of age. Proliferation of the cells within the prostate gland leads to the formation of nodules; these nodules are typically located in the transitional zone of the prostate, which surrounds the urethra. Further enlargement of the nodules results in compression of the urethra, causing frequent urination and urinary urgency. Alpha-adrenergic receptor antagonists, or alpha blockers, are commonly used to treat BPH; they work by relaxing the smooth muscle of both the prostate and the bladder to lessen some of the pressure on the urethra caused by the hyperplastic nodules. In addition to alpha blockers, 5-alpha-reductase inhibitors may also help to relieve the symptoms of BPH by stemming the growth of the prostate gland over time. Eventually, if the urethra becomes compressed enough so that the flow of urine is completely blocked, resulting in urinary retention, surgical intervention may be required.

Endometriosis:

Endometriosis is the growth of endometrial tissue outside of the endometrial cavity; it may occur on the serosal surface of the uterus or ovaries, in the abdominal cavity, or even as far away as the lungs and brain (though this is rare). It is a debilitating condition for those patients that suffer from it, and there is no cure for the disease. Medications may help relieve some or all of the symptoms, however. For pain relief, NSAIDs are commonly used; prescription narcotics may be necessary to relieve pain associated with more severe cases. Avoiding estrogens can also control symptoms, as estrogen stimulates the growth of endometrial tissue; progesterone therapy may be indicated as well, as progesterone has the opposite effect of estrogen. Oral contraceptive therapy, taken without the placebo pills, is also effective in treating endometriosis, because it eliminates menstruation. Prevention of ovulation (creating a menopause-like state) can be achieved through use of a gonadotropin-releasing hormone (GnRH) agonist such as leuprolide.

Rho(D) immune globulin (human) injection:

Rho(D) immune globulin (human) is an immunoglobulin (antibody) injection that contains immunoglobulin G (IgG) antibodies (the only class of antibody that can pass from the mother's blood through the placenta to the fetal circulation) against the D (or RhD) antigen on red blood cells. The purpose of the injection is to prevent the mother from creating antibodies against the blood of her fetus, which may result in hemolytic disease of the newborn (HDN). If the mother is Rh negative, and the fetus is Rh positive, fetal red cells that enter the maternal circulation can cause the mother to produce anti-Rh antibodies; these antibodies can then cross the placenta and destroy the red cells in the fetal circulation, causing anemia, jaundice, kernicterus (bilirubin deposits in the central nervous system), and even death. When a small amount of anti-Rh is injected into the mother, it will bind any circulating fetal cells and destroy them before the mother can produce mass amounts of antibodies.

Gastrointestinal pharmacotherapeutics

Ulcerative colitis:

Ulcerative colitis (UC) is a disease of the colon characterized by chronic inflammation, resulting in deep ulcers that involve the entire wall of the colon (transmural inflammation). Surgical resection of the colon is typically curative of the disease; however, preservation of the colon may be possible by controlling the disease with medication. Aminosalicylates, such as sulfasalazine and mesalazine, have resulted in marked improvement in patients with less severe disease. Steroids, such as prednisone, prednisolone, and hydrocortisone, are also somewhat effective in controlling UC, though the side effects of corticosteroids are somewhat undesirable. In patients with more severe UC, reasonable relief from symptoms may be achieved through low doses of some of the relatively mild chemotherapeutic drugs, including methotrexate, mercaptopurine, and azathioprine. Immunosuppressive therapy with tacrolimus (a drug commonly used to prevent rejection of transplanted solid organs) can also decrease inflammation.

Hepatitis C:

Hepatitis C is a chronic viral infection of the liver that is transferred through the blood of an infected individual; unlike hepatitis A and hepatitis B, there is no vaccination for hepatitis C. With treatment, the viral load can be eliminated in approximately half of those individuals infected with the disease. The treatment regimen consists of interferon-alpha injections in conjunction with ribavirin, an anti-viral medication. The regimen is extensive, lasting from 24 to 48 weeks; this, combined with the notorious, sometimes debilitating side effects of interferon therapy, adversely affects patient compliance. It is important that the patient follow through with the treatment, and it is also important that the treatment begin as soon as possible; noncompliance and a lag period between infection and treatment both result in an increase in viral load. The greater the viral load, the less likely that the patient will respond well to treatment.

Gastroesophageal reflux disease:

Gastroesophageal reflux disease (GERD) is a disease in which the mucosal lining of the esophagus is damaged because of reflux of acid from the stomach into the esophagus. The disease causes the symptom known as "heartburn," among other symptoms, and there are a variety of drugs that are used to treat the disease. The first group of drugs is the proton pump inhibitors (PPIs); these drugs alleviate the symptoms of GERD by inhibiting the production of stomach acid. A drug called sucralfate is also used to treat GERD, but by a different mechanism; sucralfate is what is known as a coating agent, meaning that it helps to form a protective layer over the esophageal mucosa. A group of drugs called "promotility" drugs are sort of a last line of defense for individuals who do not respond well to PPIs. Promotility drugs (such as metoclopramide and ondansetron) are typically used as antinausea medications; they tighten the lower esophageal sphincter and promote quicker emptying of the gastric contents.

Hematology and oncology pharmacotherapeutics

Breast cancer:

Tamoxifen is a drug known as a selective estrogen receptor modulator. It has seen great success in the treatment of breast cancers that are estrogen receptor positive; ER+ tumors require estrogen to grow. When the drug is administered (as a prodrug, in actuality), it is metabolized by the liver; its metabolites then bind to estrogen receptors on the tumor cells so that estrogen cannot bind, which in turn stops the tumor from growing. Tamoxifen is typically an adjuvant therapy, meaning that it is given after the primary therapy (e.g., chemotherapy, radiation) in an effort to prevent recurrence. The drug is also given to patients who are considered to be at risk for developing ER+ breast cancer in an effort to prevent the disease.

Anemias:

Erythropoietin (EPO) is a hormone produced by the kidneys (and, to a lesser extent, the liver) that stimulates the production of red blood cells. Because the kidneys produce the majority of the hormone, damage to the kidneys can result in anemia. For this reason, erythropoietin is used therapeutically to treat anemia caused by chronic renal failure. Erythropoietin is also common in treating chemotherapy patients suffering from anemia secondary to bone marrow ablation by chemotherapeutic drugs. Erythropoietin has been used to increase red cell production in patients suffering from anemia of chronic disease, which is a complication of longstanding illnesses such as heart failure, liver failure, and autoimmune diseases.

Chronic myelogenous leukemia:

Chronic myelogenous leukemia (CML) is a myeloproliferative disorder in which there is an uncontrolled production of mature granulocytes (the white blood cells associated with fighting bacterial, fungal, and parasitic infections) by the bone marrow. The disease is unique in that it is associated with a specific chromosomal abnormality, a translocation of chromosomes 9 and 22. The translocation of these 2 chromosomes results in the formation of a protein called BCR/abl, an active tyrosine kinase protein; this protein is responsible for the uncontrolled production of granulocytes. To stop this overproduction, a drug called imatinib, a tyrosine kinase inhibitor, was developed to target the BCR/abl protein. Imatinib binds to the ATP binding site on the BCR/abl protein and halts the phosphorylation of tyrosine, making it inactive. The drug has proven to be very successful in treating CML.

Immunology pharmacotherapeutics

HIV infection:

Although the components of the drug "cocktail" used to treat individuals with HIV infection and AIDS is hotly contested, and there is no perfect combination of drugs, there is one drug that most will agree should be included in any treatment regimen for the disease, and that is AZT, or zidovudine. AZT is an antiretroviral drug that works by inhibiting the action of an enzyme called reverse transcriptase, which is the enzyme that is necessary to make DNA from RNA. Without being able to form DNA, the virus cannot infect host cells. The downside of AZT is that it does not work forever, as the virus eventually develops resistance to the drug. AZT therapy is particularly effective in preventing the virus from being passed from mother to child, and it is given prophylactically to individuals who may have been exposed to the virus.

Systemic lupus erythematosus:

Systemic lupus erythematosus (SLE) is an autoimmune disease in which the body produces antibodies to its own tissues (especially the kidneys, skin, heart, joints, and blood vessels), causing inflammation and resultant damage to the tissue (which causes a subsequent decrease in the function of the tissue/organ). There is no cure for the disease, and so treatment is aimed at controlling symptoms. Aspirin, ibuprofen, and acetaminophen may be prescribed for pain. Steroids such as prednisone are an integral part of treatment in that they help to reduce inflammation; immunosuppressive and cytotoxic drugs such as cyclophosphamide also help to reduce inflammation by suppressing those cells that produce antibodies. Hydroxychloroquine, an antimalarial drug, has also been shown to improve joint and dermatologic symptoms.

Immunosuppresion:

Tacrolimus (sometimes referred to as FK506) is a non-antibiotic macrolide drug used for its immunosuppressive ability. The drug works by binding to the FK506 binding protein; this inhibits the transcription of IL-2 (a cytokine that activates lymphocytes) and blocks the transmission of signals between T cells. By disabling IL-2 transcription and T-cell signaling, tacrolimus greatly compromises the body's immune response. For this reason, the drug is widely used to guard against rejection of transplanted solid organs (e.g., liver, kidney, lungs). Although the drug was developed to prevent post-transplant rejection, it has more recently been used (rather experimentally, however) to treat ulcerative colitis. A topical form of the drug has also shown some promise in the treatment of eczema.

Anaphylaxis:

Anaphylaxis is a severe, systemic hypersensitivity (allergic) reaction that is classified as a type I hypersensitivity. If an individual suffering from an anaphylactic reaction is not treated immediately, death is likely. The systemic symptoms of anaphylaxis (hypotension, difficulty breathing, and angioedema) result from the release of large amounts of histamine from mast cells. When released into the bloodstream, histamine causes the bronchioles to constrict; it also causes vasodilation (relaxation of the blood vessels, resulting in a decrease in blood pressure) and leakage of fluids into the surrounding tissue (resulting in edema and a further decline in blood pressure). When an individual is suffering from an anaphylactic reaction, treatment with epinephrine is the best way to stabilize the patient. Epinephrine is a powerful vasoconstrictor, and an equally powerful bronchodilator; it also increases heart rate and stroke volume to counteract the shock that occurs as a result of the anaphylactic reaction.

Rheumatoid arthritis:

Rheumatoid arthritis (RA) is an autoimmune disease causing chronic inflammation of the joints; there is no cure for the disease, and treatment is palliative. Steroids such as prednisone and NSAIDs are used to reduce inflammation in the joints. Methotrexate, a drug with immunosuppressive abilities, is also used to reduce inflammation. Hydroxychloroquine, an antimalarial drug, has been shown to improve the inflammation that is a hallmark of autoimmune diseases, including RA and SLE. Sulfasalazine, which is classified as a disease-modifying anti-rheumatic drug (DMARD), also helps to inhibit the inflammatory process, though the mechanism is unknown. Tumor necrosis factor (TNF) inhibitors halt inflammation by inactivating TNF, a proinflammatory chemical released by lymphocytes.

Musculoskeletal pharmacotherapeutics

Gout:

Gout is a metabolic disease in which uric acid crystals form and deposit in and around the joints, causing subsequent painful inflammation. One of the first drugs developed for the treatment of gout was colchicine, a derivative of the autumn crocus plant. Although colchicine has fallen out of favor somewhat, it still may be prescribed for the disease, and the side effects of the treatment should be recognized. Colchicine works by inhibiting both the movement of granulocytes (which are responsible for cell-mediated inflammation) and the deposition of uric acid crystals. Colchicine also has the ability to inhibit mitosis, which results in many of the unpleasant side effects; these include diarrhea, vomiting, kidney failure, and bone marrow damage leading to anemia, leucopenia, and thrombocytopenia.

Osteoporosis:

Osteoporosis is a disease in which the density of bone is decreased, leading to a greater risk of pathologic bone fracture. A daily calcium supplement, taken with a vitamin D supplement, can help to increase the mineral density of the bone. Drugs that inhibit osteoclasts, the cells responsible for bone resorption (breakdown), are effective in preventing further bone loss; these drugs include calcitonin (a hormone naturally produced by the thyroid gland) and the bisphosphonates. The hormone estrogen is known to increase the formation of new bone, thereby increasing bone density, and is another reason that hormone replacement therapy is helpful for postmenopausal women.

Psychosocial pharmacotherapeutics

Clozapine:

Clozapine is a second-generation antipsychotic drug that is used to treat schizophrenic patients with refractory disease (meaning that the disease does not respond to other treatments). Although the drug has proven to be a great treatment for refractory schizophrenia, its use must be carefully monitored, because it has a potentially life-threatening side effect called agranulocytosis. Agranulocytosis, or a lack of granulocytes in the blood, means that the patient does not have the ability to fight off bacterial infections. This side effect occurs in between 1% and 2% of patients taking clozapine, which is not an insignificant number. For this reason, the FDA requires that patients being treated with the drug submit to mandatory weekly blood testing so that granulocyte levels can be monitored, and the drug can be discontinued if levels begin to drop.

Haloperidol:
Haloperidol is a first-generation, or typical, antipsychotic drug that is used in the treatment of schizophrenia, acute psychosis, mania, and delirium. A more accurate classification of the drug is as a neuroleptic, meaning that it works by blocking dopamine receptors in the brain, specifically in the limbic system, which includes the hippocampus and controls behavior and emotions. Because haloperidol is such a strong anti-dopaminergic drug, it has untoward side effects related to motor function. These side effects are referred to as extrapyramidal effects, and can be disfiguring and even permanent, depending on the amount and length of treatment. Examples of extrapyramidal side effects include dystonia (abnormal, awkward posturing, muscle cramping and spasms), akathisia (internal restlessness and anxiety), bradykinesia (slow movements), and even akinesia (the physical inability to move).

Serotonin syndrome:
The serotonin syndrome is a group of symptoms that occur as a result of overstimulation of serotonin receptors in the central and peripheral nervous systems; it may also be referred to as serotonin toxicity. The clinical picture for serotonin syndrome includes tachycardia, hypertension, hyperthermia, diaphoresis, shivering, tremor, headache, nausea, diarrhea, agitation, and confusion. A patient suffering from serotonin syndrome may exhibit all of these symptoms, or only a few, depending on the level of stimulation of the serotonin receptors. Patients with severe hyperthermia and shock may become acidotic and progress to rhabdomyolysis, renal failure, and seizure. Drugs that have been implicated in contributing to the serotonin syndrome include MDMA (ecstasy), SSRIs, monoamine oxidase inhibitors (MAOIs), cocaine, amphetamines, LSD, lithium, and even certain antibiotics such as linezolid and erythromycin.

Lithium:
Lithium exists as an ion in the form of an alkali metal; combined with other elements to form a lithium salt, it is used as a mood-stabilizing drug for the treatment of both the depressive and (to a greater extent) manic phases of bipolar disorder. Lithium works both by decreasing the amount of circulating norepinephrine (a hormone that increases heart rate, blood glucose levels, and alertness) and increasing production of serotonin. Lithium is somewhat unique in

that the therapeutic level of the drug is very close to the toxic level; for this reason, blood lithium levels must be carefully monitored to ensure that the patient is within the therapeutic window. Because lithium causes some degree of dysregulation of both water and sodium, patients taking lithium can become dehydrated. It is important that patients remain hydrated and maintain appropriate sodium intake. In addition to regular monitoring of lithium levels, patients should be monitored for both kidney and thyroid function.

Morphine:
Morphine is an opioid drug whose main benefit is pain relief. Because it is such a strong pain reliever, morphine is often used to treat the pain associated with cancer, kidney stones, sickle cell crisis, heart attack, bone fracture, and surgical procedures. Along with its strong pain-relieving ability, however, morphine also carries with it a strong addictive component. Patients using morphine to treat pain often find themselves addicted, even after a short period of time. Individuals who have been taking morphine for long periods of time are much more susceptible to the withdrawal symptoms, as dependence increases over time. Withdrawal symptoms include diarrhea, sweating, restlessness, insomnia, tremor, nausea, vomiting, hot flashes, and bone and muscle pain.

Activated charcoal:
Activated charcoal (or activated carbon) is used in the treatment of patients with acute poisoning associated with ingestion of a chemical or drug. Syrup of ipecac is another method to rid the body of poison, although it causes the individual to vomit; vomiting of a toxic substance can lead to further damage as the substance exits the body, and it also has no effect on substances that have already entered the intestines. Activated charcoal, on the other hand, works by adsorption, meaning that the toxin attaches to the surface of the charcoal molecules, reducing the potency of the toxins. The charcoal (a fine black powder) is usually administered either orally (by giving the patient a solution to drink) or through a nasogastric tube.

Clinical Therapeutics

Nutrition

Starvation:
When the body is deprived of nutrition, it must rely on its own energy stores; the energy stores available for use are glycogen (stored in the liver and skeletal muscle), fat (adipose tissue), and protein from skeletal and smooth muscle. In the beginning stages of starvation, once blood glucose has been depleted and insulin levels drop, the body will release glucose stores from the liver by breaking down glycogen (a process called glycogenolysis). After approximately 24 hours, when liver stores have been depleted, the body manufactures glucose (called gluconeogenesis) through catabolism of protein. Progression of starvation leads to breakdown of fat (called lipolysis), which results in the formation of ketones and ketoacids. As the body

adapts to these physiologic changes, the caloric need decreases, because the metabolic rate slows in an effort to conserve energy stores.

Stressed starvation vs. simple starvation: When the body is stressed, the physiological changes that result from starvation are altered because of the response of stress hormones such as cortisol, as well as epinephrine and norepinephrine. Cortisol, a hormone released during stress, causes blood glucose levels to remain elevated through increased gluconeogenesis (breakdown of proteins to form glucose). The persistent high level of glucose leads to insulin resistance, which further perpetuates the high blood glucose level. In addition, the stimulation of gluconeogenesis by cortisol results in a depletion of protein, which is why stressed starvation may also be referred to as hypoalbuminemic malnutrition. Because gluconeogenesis is continuous, fat stores are not used up as they are during simple starvation; this leads to a wasting of muscle mass without loss of fat stores, so that the individual may still be perceived as "obese" although he or she is not receiving enough nutrition.

24-hour recall:

When the nurse practitioner is interviewing a patient and wants to gain a basic knowledge or understanding of the patient's nutritional state, he or she can incorporate questioning about food intake into the history and physical. Although a licensed dietitian may be able to elicit a more comprehensive food history, it is important to the overall clinical picture for the nurse practitioner to have a working knowledge of the patient's diet. To get a rough idea, the NP may conduct a 24-hour recall, meaning that he or she asks what foods and beverages have been consumed by the patient in the past 24 hours. Of course, this may or may not be representative of the patient's regular diet (and the patient may choose not to mention certain foods that he or she thinks are "bad"), but it can be useful information to have.

Daily food guidelines:

The Basic Four and the Food Pyramid are both guidelines established to aid individuals when making food choices; they are meant to help individuals structure a diet in order to accommodate the daily recommended allowances for each food group. The Basic Four is a less comprehensive outline; it provides the bare minimum nutritional requirements so that the individual does not become deficient in any nutritional area. The Basic Four recommends the following daily servings: 2 servings of dairy, 4 servings of simple carbohydrates (breads and cereals), and 2 servings each of meats, fruits, and vegetables. The Food Pyramid, on the other hand, is more comprehensive, recommending a daily intake of 2 to 3 servings of dairy, 6 to 11 servings of carbohydrates, 2 to 4 servings of fruits, 3 to 5 servings of meats, and 2 to 3 servings of vegetables. Both guidelines recommend sparing intake of both fats and sugars.

Anthropometry:

Anthropometry is defined as the measurement of either a part of the body or the entire body; basic examples include height and weight measurements. Weight is an important measurement when determining the caloric requirements of an individual; the ideal weight is usually determined based on the individual's height. Of course, no two people are alike, and the ideal weight for one may not be the ideal weight for another. Perhaps the most accurate method to date for calculating ideal body weight is the body mass index (BMI). BMI is typically calculated by dividing the weight (in kilograms) by the square of the height (in meters). A BMI greater than 25 is typically considered to be overweight, while a BMI greater than 30 is considered obese. The Hamwi equation provides a rough estimate of ideal weight; a 5 ft woman is considered to be 100 lbs; for each inch over 5 ft, 5 pounds are added, so that a woman measuring 5'7" has an ideal weight of 135 lbs.

Body fat distribution: Another example of an anthropometric measurement is the waist to hip ratio; to calculate this ratio, the individual divides the circumference of his or her waist (measured at the level of the umbilicus) by the circumference or his or her hips (measured where the buttocks are at their widest point). This helps to determine the distribution of an individual's body fat, which is an important indicator of health. An individual who tends to store fat around the abdomen, arms, and back ("apple-shaped" body type), for example, is at a greater risk of cardiovascular disease and diabetes than is an individual who accumulates fat in the thighs and buttocks ("pear-shaped" body type). It has been shown that individuals with excess abdominal (visceral) fat usually accumulate fat in that area because of a growing insulin resistance, which can lead to diabetes and cardiovascular problems. For women, the ideal waist to hip ratio is less than 0.8, and for men less than 1.0.

Nutritional status:

There are several markers of nutritional status. To determine the status of protein levels and consumption, the best markers are albumin, prealbumin, and transferrin. Albumin is the most abundant of all the serum proteins, and is important to the regulation of many of the body's physiologic functions; for this reason, it is often considered a "homeostasis" protein. Low levels of albumin (and prealbumin) can indicate poor nutrition. However, the levels of these proteins are also influenced by many other factors, including hydration, renal function, and liver function; the presence of a malignancy will also have an effect on serum protein levels. In the instance that other factors can be ruled out, low albumin (called hypoalbuminemia) is a fairly good indicator of poor nutritional status. Transferrin, another serum protein, is a good indicator of improving nutrition; transferrin levels rise fairly quickly when an individual begins to restore protein levels.

Screening tools: Assessing the nutritional status of the hospital inpatient is an important part of forming a care plan. The 2 screening tools that are most commonly used are the Subjective Global Assessment (SGA) and the Prognostic Nutritional Index (PNI). The SGA provides a nutritional assessment based on both the patient history and current symptoms. The patient is asked about any changes in weight, and is also asked questions about his or her diet. The presence of symptoms that may lead to weight loss and poor nutritional status, such as diarrhea, nausea, and vomiting, as well as water retention (edema) and muscle wasting (cachexia), is also included in the SGA. The PNI is also used as an indicator of malnutrition, and is especially helpful in determining how well a patient will recover from surgery; the PNI assesses nutritional status through the measurement of serum proteins such as albumin and transferrin, combined with a skinfold measurement and a cutaneous hypersensitivity test (as an indicator of immune function).

Vitamin D:

Vitamin D is necessary for the intestinal absorption of both calcium and phosphorus, which is the reason that milk is fortified with vitamin D. It also aids in the reabsorption of calcium at the distal convoluted tubule in the kidney, and it promotes bone formation. Vitamin D is actually a prohormone called ergocalciferol, and requires ultraviolet light for synthesis into its active form, called cholecalciferol. Deficiency of vitamin D (whether due to lack of ingestion, lack of exposure to sunlight, or both) results in softening of the bones because of reabsorption of calcium and phosphorus, which form the mineral matrix of bone. In children, this bone softening is called rickets, and in adults it is called osteomalacia. Vitamin D deficiency may also contribute to osteoporosis. Symptoms of osteomalacia include bone pain (starting in the back and legs, then involving the chest and arms), muscle weakness, and fatigue. Nausea, vomiting, diarrhea, headache, and soft tissue calcification are all indicative of vitamin D toxicity.

Enteral and parenteral support:

Enteral nutrition is a method of providing nutrition to a patient through a tube; the tube may be placed in either the nose (a nasogastric tube), the stomach (a percutaneous endoscopic gastrostomy [PEG] tube), or the small bowel (a percutaneous endoscopic jejunal [J] tube). When the tube has been placed, nutrition can be administered through the tube and absorbed by the patient's digestive system. Various enteric formulas exist, and the choice is dependent on the nutritional requirements of the patient. Parenteral nutrition (also called total parenteral nutrition [TPN]) is a method of providing nutrition that completely bypasses the digestive system by administering nutrition through an intravenous line. Enteral support is the preferred method of providing nutrition, although in patients suffering from some compromise of the gastrointestinal tract, parenteral nutrition is the only option.

Complications of parenteral nutrition: Although parenteral nutrition is a great method for providing nutrition to severely ill patients who cannot tolerate enteral support, it should be avoided unless absolutely necessary because there are many risk factors associated with this type of nutritional support. Most of the problems that occur during treatment with parenteral nutrition are related to the indwelling catheter; it is a common site for infection, and, in the compromised patient, sepsis is both more likely and more dangerous. Catheters may also move or dislodge, causing discomfort and other problems; they can become clogged, and clots can form and then break off, resulting in thrombosis. Air bubbles in the tubing can enter the bloodstream, causing an air embolus. The patient may also have problems tolerating the nutritional supplements, and it can be difficult to control glucose levels as well.

Determining caloric requirements:
When an individual requires hospitalization for a critical illness, his or her caloric requirements must be determined so that normal body function is maintained, and so that recovery is as quick as possible. There are many factors that must be considered when attempting to determine the requirements of an ill patient. First, the age of the patient is important. If the patient is a growing child or adolescent, he or she will have very different nutritional requirements than an elderly individual would have. Also to be considered is the physical and nutritional status of the patient, independent of the illness. A patient who is normally very active would have different requirements than an overweight, sedentary individual. Along the same lines, comorbidities, such as diabetes and atherosclerosis, need to be considered, as well as overall stress levels of the patient.

Harris Benedict equation: The Harris Benedict equation is a useful tool when determining the caloric requirements necessary for the critically ill patient. The goal of the equation is to determine the resting energy expenditure of the patient; that is, what is the baseline energy level that is required to maintain physiological function. The equation considers the factors of age, weight, and height when calculating caloric requirements. For women, the resting energy expenditure is calculated as 655 + (9.6 x weight in kilograms) + (1.7 x height in centimeters) – (4.7 x age in years). For men, resting energy expenditure is calculated as 66 + (13.7 x weight in kilograms) + (5 x height in centimeters) – (6.8 x age in years). Additional modifications can be made to the equation to accommodate differences in activity and stress levels.

Exercise:
Exercise is important for overall cardiovascular health; lack of exercise has been associated with various health problems, including high blood pressure, atherosclerosis, and type II diabetes. Exercise can be beneficial for diabetic patients, although special precautions must be taken, because there are associated risks as well. Type I diabetics will see an improvement in both cardiovascular function and overall health and well-being; however, exercise can make it more difficult to control blood sugar levels. The type I diabetic should never begin an exercise regimen unless his or her disease is under control. Type I diabetics will also see an improvement in cardiovascular function, in addition to weight loss, which (along with proper diet) may slow or even reverse the diabetic state. The type II diabetic should be evaluated by a physician before beginning any exercise plan; ischemia, repetition injury, trauma, and heat exhaustion are among the risks for these patients.

Obesity:
Obesity is usually defined based on either BMI or ideal body weight as calculated using the Hamwi equation. Using BMI as a reference, obesity is defined as a BMI greater than 27, while a BMI greater than 30 is considered severely (or morbidly) obese. Using an ideal body weight calculation, weight greater than 20% above the ideal body weight is considered obese, while weight greater than 40% above the ideal body weight is considered to be severely obese. Although these are good guidelines to use when evaluating an overweight individual, other factors must be considered. Factors that have been shown to correlate to obesity include lack of physical activity, poor or inappropriate diet, genetics, and economic class.

Rehabilitation

Rehabilitation is an area of health care that is dedicated to helping patients improve and/or restore functions and abilities after a disease or injury. Although rehabilitation is usually thought of in relation to physical therapy (which is one of the many areas of rehabilitation), it also encompasses drug and alcohol rehabilitation, as well as occupational therapy for physically and mentally ill patients. The general goals of all types of rehabilitation include an improvement in overall function; the promotion of independence, satisfaction, and well-being; and the preservation of the individual's self esteem in the face of illness or debilitating disease or injury.

Activities of daily living:
Activities of daily living (ADLs) are a group of activities that are used to evaluate a patient's return to normal function; these are activities that the patient had performed on a daily basis before hospitalization, and will be expected to perform once he or she has completed rehabilitation. The rate at which the patient accomplishes these activities, in addition to the level of independence maintained by the patient when performing the activities, can help caregivers determine the amount of rehabilitation required, and can also be used to monitor the progress of the patient during the rehabilitation process. ADLs are grouped into 3 different areas: personal and physical, instrumental, and occupational.

The first group of ADLs, the physical or personal group, contains those daily activities that relate to the patient's ability to take care of him or herself. Included in this group are activities related to health management, nutritional needs, elimination of bladder and bowel contents, exercise, self-esteem, coping/stress management, cognitive abilities, communication, sexual health and ability, and relationship roles. The second group of ADLs, the instrumental group, contains activities such as shopping, answering the phone, and other activities that involve leaving home. The third group, occupational activities, includes activities that are required of being a parent, husband, or wife, as well as those required on the job.

Need for rehabilitation:
There are some diseases, illnesses, and injuries that almost always require rehabilitation at some point during their course; in these cases, rehabilitation may be initiated before the patient even leaves the hospital to be transferred to a rehabilitation facility. It is important to know which diseases usually require rehabilitation, because the sooner evaluation and rehabilitation are initiated, the better the patient's chance of recovery. The following are diseases, illnesses, and injuries that commonly require rehabilitation: AIDS, amyotrophic lateral sclerosis (ALS), limb amputation, traumatic or ischemic brain injury, spinal cord injury, burns, Guillain-Barré syndrome, hip or knee replacement, multiple sclerosis (MS), and most types of cancer.

Patient's potential for rehabilitation:
There are various factors that are considered when assessing a patient to determine whether he or she will benefit from rehabilitation. A patient with the inability to perform any of the ADLs will automatically be considered for rehabilitation; at this point, however, other factors must be considered. First and foremost is whether or not the patient has a desire to improve his or her functions through rehabilitation; if the patient is not interested in improvement, the rehabilitation potential is poor. If the patient wants to improve function and increase independence, the potential for rehabilitation is greater. Another factor is whether or not the patient has support at home; even if the patient improves greatly during his or her rehabilitation stay, he or she will still most likely need some support at home. If the patient has no support at home, rehabilitation may eventually fail.

Interventions:
When a patient is to be considered for rehabilitation, he or she must undergo a rather extensive evaluation in order to increase the likelihood that he or she will succeed during rehabilitation. This process of evaluation, which includes various interventions, should take place in the early stages of illness, when the patient is still in the hospital. The goal is to forestall any secondary complications that may inhibit the rehabilitation process. These interventions include health management, in which the patient and family are educated about his or her disease(s); nutritional status assessment and support; initiation of bowel and bladder management in order to prevent infection; exercises; assessment of cognitive function; and education involving self-esteem, relationship roles, sexual activity, and coping mechanisms.

Rehabilitation settings:
There are various kinds of rehabilitation settings, depending on the needs of the patient. Once the need for rehabilitation has been determined, and the patient has been evaluated regarding specific rehabilitation needs, he or she can be placed in an appropriate rehabilitation setting. A long-term acute care hospital is a rehabilitation facility that is best for patients who are physically and psychologically stable, but are receiving medical treatment such as dialysis or ventilation, and thus require

medical support. A subacute care unit is appropriate for patients who require more limited treatment, such as cancer patients. A comprehensive inpatient rehabilitation facility is just what the name suggests; it addresses the needs of a broad range of different patients, from burn victims to amputees. The comprehensive rehabilitation center has a "team" of medical specialists that includes a rehabilitation medicine physician, nurses trained in rehabilitation, occupational therapists, physical therapists, social workers, and speech-language pathologists. Outpatient rehab is designed for the high-functioning patient who can return home after rehab sessions.

Occupational therapy

Occupational therapy is defined as the use of creative activities in the treatment of disabled individuals, whether they are disabled physically or mentally. The purpose of occupational therapy is to provide disabled individuals with the skills that are necessary to live life as fully and independently as possible; after completion of occupational therapy, the individual should be able to perform at his or her maximum potential. The occupational therapist will typically provide the patient with interventions tailored to his or her disability. The OT will also visit the patient's home and/or place of employment in order to assess potential problems and provide adaptive solutions. As part of occupational therapy, the patient will receive regular assessments of his or her skills, as well as specific training. The occupational therapist is also responsible for educating the patient's family, caretakers, friends, and coworkers.

Philosophy:

The philosophy of occupational therapy is based on the idea that occupation (meaning, loosely, either an activity or activities in which an individual engages) is a basic human need, one that is important to an individual's health and overall well-being in that it is in and of itself therapeutic in nature. The basic assumptions of occupational therapy are based on the idea of occupational therapy as stated by its creator, William Rush Dunton. Dunton states that occupational therapy is a human need because an individual's occupation has an effect on his or her health and general well-being. It creates structure in the individual's life, and allows for him or her to manage and organize time. Another assumption is that individuals have different sets of values, and therefore will value different occupations; for each person, however, the occupation that he or she chooses is meaningful to him or her.

Areas of practice:

Although occupational therapy is an important part of the overall rehabilitation process for hospitalized individuals, it is also beneficial in other areas, because occupational therapy deals not only with physical disabilities, but with emotional and cognitive disabilities as well. Occupational therapy as related to physical disabilities may be practiced in outpatient clinics, pediatric hospitals or units, acute care rehabilitation facilities, and long-term, or comprehensive, inpatient rehabilitation centers. Occupational therapy as related to mental disabilities may be practiced in mental health clinics, acute and long-term psychiatric hospitals, prisons, and gateway or halfway houses. Occupational therapists may also work at schools, childcare facilities, workplaces, or shelters, or they may even work with individuals in their own homes.

Clinical decision making

Medical reasoning:
Medical reasoning refers to the process by which clinicians gather data and information about a patient, and, using those data, arrive at a diagnosis and treatment plan.

Diagnostic and **therapeutic reasoning**:
Diagnostic reasoning and therapeutic reasoning are subsets of medical reasoning; diagnostic reasoning is the information that is used to determine the most likely diagnosis, while therapeutic reasoning is the information used to determine what the best treatment is for that particular patient suffering from that particular disease.

Therapeutic uncertainty:
While the patient is undergoing treatment, it is necessary for the clinician to evaluate the patient's response to treatment on a regular basis. If it is not clear whether the patient is improving, or whether another treatment might be more beneficial, a degree of therapeutic uncertainty is introduced. There is also therapeutic uncertainty when the clinician is trying to decide which treatment option to use if the first treatment fails.

Diagnostic uncertainty:
Diagnosis and subsequent treatment are not easily arrived at for every patient because every patient is different. The clinical presentation of a heart attack, for example, may include severe chest pain, sweating, and nausea for one patient, and may have very mild, almost unnoticeable symptoms in another. Diagnostic uncertainty is especially prominent when dealing with diseases that have nonspecific symptoms; in these cases, it is important that the clinician recognize which of the possible diagnoses are life-threatening, and which are not. Ruling out the life-threatening possibilities should be higher on the clinician's list of priorities than the nonlife-threatening ones. Diagnostic testing, and subsequent treatment options, should also be evaluated according to the risks and benefits to the patient.

Clinical uncertainty:
Although the degree of uncertainty is somewhat dependent on the patient, the clinical setting can have an influence on the degree of uncertainty that the clinician is likely to encounter. For example, a clinic, such as a dermatology clinic, is a setting in which the degree of uncertainty is likely to be low; this is because the clinic is nonemergent, and because the clinic treats a specific, limited group of diseases with

which the clinicians are very familiar. An urgent care clinic would fall somewhere in the middle, because although there is a wider range of diagnostic possibility, life-threatening emergencies are rarely encountered. An emergency room or a trauma center, on the other hand, sees a high degree of uncertainty; the clinicians see a wide range of diagnostic possibilities, and are expected to work at a fast pace.

Intuitive decision-making

When a clinician makes an intuitive decision, he or she is making a decision not necessarily based on fact, but more so because it feels like the right decision. Of course, in most cases, one would not want a doctor making decisions this way, although in certain cases (say, a choice between 2 different types of treatment, each of which has the same general risks, or when all other options have been exhausted), it may be necessary. Although these decisions are not based on an analysis of the facts, there is something to be said about the so-called "gut instinct," which years of training and experience can hone. These decisions are made without spending a lot of time on the process of decision making; though they are based on experience, the clinician may suffer some degree of anxiety about the decision and its outcome.

Analytical decision making

An analytical decision is one that is made after a systematic review and analysis of all factors involved in the decision; concentration and awareness are important in the analytical decision-making process. In contrast with an intuitive decision, the analytical decision takes longer to make, because it is not automatic. The analysis is based on an in-depth look at all factors, and is based on scientific evidence (in other words, it is based on the outcomes of previous similar situations). Because an analytical decision is based on scientific evidence and facts, the outcome of the decision has a high predictive value; this means that by looking at previous outcomes, it is possible to predict the current outcome. Because the clinician has so carefully reviewed all factors, he or she will most likely not experience the emotional anxiety associated with an intuitive decision.

Clinical decision-making process

Although one would like to think that there isn't much variation in the clinical decision-making process, this simply is not true. The process, of course, will differ depending on the patient, the differential diagnosis, and the clinician. First, let's start with the clinician. The way that the clinician conducts the clinical decision-making process is influenced by the knowledge base of the clinician, as well as the level of his experience, the ability he possesses to think both critically and creatively, and the confidence that he has in his ability to make educated decisions. The acuity level of the patient is also a factor in the clinical decision-making process, as is the length of the differential. A time stressor is placed on the clinician when the condition of the patient is critical, and when there are more diseases that must be eliminated from the differential. An element of stress may also exist if the clinician has a high number of patients, especially if he has multiple high-acuity patients.

External stressors:
Aside from time (or lack thereof), there are other external or environmental stressors that may have an effect on the clinical decision-making process. One of these stressors is inadequate staffing. If the department does not have enough staff to handle the workload, or if there are not enough experienced staff members to help the less-experienced staff members, this can cause problems with the decision-making process, both by adding a time stressor, and by not providing enough resources for the staff. Another stressor that has an effect on the clinical decision-making process is the presence of strained interpersonal relationships; strained relationships may occur between 2 or more nurses, between physicians, or between nurses and physicians. Whatever the combination, a strained relationship between individuals who should be working together can negatively impact decision making.

Safety:
In 2005, Ebright et al published a study of factors related to safety and the decision-making ability of the nurse. Every clinical decision made by the nurse has an effect on the safety of the patient, and therefore any factor that influences the nurse's decision-making ability may adversely affect the patient. Ebright at al identified the following factors that influence decision-making and patient safety: knowledge base, attention, barriers to care, number of tasks, missing essential information, and behaviors that are not encouraging of productive thought. The presence of, or a change in, any of these factors can result in unnecessary harm for the patient.

Knowledge base, attention, and barriers to care: Knowledge base refers to the amount of working knowledge that is available to the practicing nurse; a new graduate, for example, will not have as broad a knowledge base as a veteran nurse. A new nurse may not be able to make confident clinical decisions, which can put the patient at risk; for this reason, it is important that there be more experienced nurses available for consultation. Attention simply refers to the amount of attention that the nurse is dedicating to the patient and his or her complaints. Attention may be compromised by any number of things; for example, maybe the nurse is preoccupied by something outside of work. This can be detrimental to the patient as well; the nurse should always devote his or her full attention to the patient. There are many barriers that may compromise the safety of the patient as well. Perhaps there are not enough beds to keep up with new admissions, or maybe no one is available for an urgent consult.

Number of tasks, missing essential information, and behaviors not encouraging of productive thought: The number of tasks assigned to a nurse can have an adverse effect both on the nurse's decision-making abilities and on the safety of the patient. If the nurse has too many things to do in too short a time, he or she will not be able to dedicate the time necessary for diagnosis, decision-making, and treatment, and the patient will suffer. If the nurse is missing information that is essential to diagnosis, such as a complete history, or a list of current medications, he or she cannot make well-informed decisions that would be best for the patient. Behaviors not encouraging of productive thought include daydreaming, multitasking, and other distractions that make it impossible for the nurse to dedicate his or her full attention to the clinical decision-making process.

Safety

Factors affecting patient safety

Ebright et al identified several factors that are common roadblocks to the delivery of safe and effective patient care. Access to supplies is one factor that influences patient safety and quality of care; an increase in the number of supply stations, and an effort to keep these stations stocked at all times, can cut the amount of time wasted on searching for or refilling supplies. In addition to the time spent running back and forth to supply stations, nurses also spent a great deal of time traveling from one patient's room to another, to the nurse's station and back, and to other locations. Assigning nurses to patients that are located near one another can help reduce time spent traveling. Distractions, interruptions, and time spent waiting for computer systems and instruments to boot up are also detrimental to patient care, though sometimes unavoidable. Nurses can make a concerted effort, however, to reduce errors in mislabeling and poor handwriting.

Patient safety assessments

There are 4 basic assessments that the nurse should make when assessing a patient's safety and identifying possible safety concerns. The first of these is the mobility assessment; different safety risks apply to patients who are mobile as opposed to those who are not. An immobile patient, for example, has a tendency to form pressure ulcers, or bedsores. The next assessment is the evaluation of the patient's level of awareness; is the patient able to communicate to the nursing staff when something is wrong? If not, certain measures should be undertaken to ensure that the nursing staff is aware of a change in the patient's condition. An extension of this assessment is determining whether the patient is in critical condition; these patients must be monitored more closely for changes. An assessment of the patient's mental status is also important, because the patient may not be able to make safe decisions on his or her own.

Administration of medication

It is extremely important that the utmost care be taken when administering medication; administering the incorrect medication, the wrong dosage, or a medication to which the patient is allergic can have disastrous consequences. A helpful way to make sure that all the bases are covered is to remember the "rights" of medication administration. First, the nurse should check to make sure that he or she has the right patient. Next, the nurse should make sure that he or she is administering the right medication. Then, the nurse should check to make sure that the dosage is correct. Making sure that the route of administration is correct is also important. Next, the nurse should make sure that the medication is being administered at the correct time. Finally, the nurse should make sure that the documentation regarding the medication administration is correct.

Increasing patient safety

Not all errors are preventable, but in the hospital setting, when errors can mean the difference between life and death, it is important that proper measures are undertaken to eliminate as many opportunities for error as possible. To prevent patient mix-ups, for instance, patients are required to wear an armband containing identification; the nurse or physician must check this identification against all orders to make sure that he or she has the correct patient. Hospital personnel should also wear an identifying tag or badge that contains the name of the employee, as well as his or her title and certification. This will help identify the employee not just to the patients but also to other employees. Another safeguard is the placement of signs on patient doors; these signs alert staff and other patients to any precautions that must be undertaken before entering the room, or while in the room (e.g., airborne precautions, fall precautions, elopement precautions).

Electronic medical records: Traditionally, the patient chart consisted of a clipboard with admission notes, progress notes, lab orders and results, and other patient information. There existed the potential for the chart to be lost or misplaced; in addition, serious errors in medication, patient identification, and ordering of tests could be attributed to a clinician's inability to decipher another clinician's handwritten notes. This one set of notes also made it difficult for other clinicians and allied health personnel in other departments to assess the patient. The advent of the electronic medical record helped to eliminate some of the problems associated with paper charts. Since the notes are entered into a computer system, illegible handwriting is no longer a source of error. The computerized system also allows clinicians in other areas of the hospital to access necessary information on patients, which improves the communication between clinicians and departments.

Health Promotion and Disease Prevention

Risk factor analysis

Neuman framework

The Neuman framework of nursing health promotion is a broad, flexible perspective that can be applied to nearly any situation that the acute care nurse may encounter in practice. The framework is based around the idea of a "client system," which may represent an individual patient, or it may represent a family, group, or entire community. In the Neuman framework, the client system is an ever-changing, open network that is constantly interacting with both the internal environment and the external environment. The role of the nurse in this framework is to identify stressors within these environments that are harming or have the potential to harm the client system. Once the nurse has identified these stressors, it is his or her job to educate the client system about them, and to help them work through them, so that the client system can maintain a healthy, balanced environment.

Risk assessment

The development of the Neuman's framework was meant to provide nursing caregivers with a guideline to help them understand the role he or she has in promoting health and well-being among individual patients and communities alike. Because each patient has individual stressors that are unique to him or her, it is necessary for the nurse to identify these stressors and tailor his or her approach to the patient (or family, or community). By identifying these unique stressors, the nurse can assess the patient's risk regarding certain diseases and illnesses. Risk factor analysis and assessment is a necessary step toward educating the patient. Once the nurse identifies these risk factors, he or she can discuss these with the patient and offer suggestions for risk reduction, starting the patient on the road to a healthier life.

<u>Primary, secondary, and tertiary prevention:</u>
Risk assessment can be divided into 3 different prevention strategies; for the nurse, this depends largely on the point at which he or she intervenes with the patient. Nurses that work in community health clinics, public health, urgent care, and primary care, for example, will most often be focused on primary and secondary prevention; the acute care nurse practitioner, on the other hand, is typically concerned with secondary and tertiary prevention. Primary prevention involves patient education concerning stressors, allowing the patient to identify and defend against them; the focus in this case is on illness prevention. If an illness is identified, secondary prevention focuses on immediate treatment and alleviation of symptoms.

Tertiary prevention focuses on the reduction of future stressors, as well as preparation of the patient to readapt to the environment.

Progression of risk assessment:

It is important for the primary care nurse practitioner (PCNP) and the acute care nurse practitioner (ACNP) to communicate with one another concerning risk assessment. The relationship becomes clear as you consider the role of each caregiver. Assume that patient X presents to his PCNP complaining of shortness of breath. The PCNP, through the history and physical examination, can narrow the differential diagnosis to a cardiac cause, and then refer the patient to cardiology. The ACNP, in reviewing the information from the PCNP, can then begin screening tests (if they have not already been done). With all of this information together (the history and physical, the risk assessment provided by the PCNP, and the test results), the ACNP can develop a treatment plan for the patient.

Person-centered care:

"Person-centered care" is a patient-care model that was developed by Allen Barbour; in his model, which is somewhat a critique of the standard medical model, he states that person-centered care "refer[s] specifically to becoming familiar with the patient's personal situation in its crucial relationship to the source of illness." The nurse's role in risk assessment as outlined by Neuman framework definitely allows room for the idea of person-centered care, because it includes a look not only at the patient's physiological stressors, but also at his or her psychologic, social, and cultural stressors. Often times these stressors are brushed aside to assess pathophysiological issues. The nurse is in a unique position in that he or she has more interaction with the patient on a personal level, and can help identify these other stressors that have just as significant an impact on the patient's illness progression and recovery.

Illness prevention:

The US Department of Health and Human Services' Guide to Clinical Preventive Services states that there are 2 important factors that must be considered above all else when evaluating a patient for preventive services. First, the nurse must consider how effective a clinical intervention will be in improving the outcome of the patient, and, second, the nurse must consider what the overall leading causes of mortality and morbidity are. The leading causes of mortality and morbidity can be assessed by population, whether it is age, sex, or some other risk-associated population. Once the patient has been assessed for the appropriate population-related risk factors, and once the nurse has determined the best intervention based on these risk factors, preventive services can be initiated.

Preventive care and health promotion:

Of late, risk assessment, preventive medicine, and health promotion have become more and more important, and the focus of numerous studies. A study by Friede et al notes that almost 70% of illness, and the social, physical, psychological, and economical burden associated with it, is preventable. This is a staggering number, and highlights the importance of prevention. Healthy People 2000 and its follow-up Healthy People 2010 were published by the US Department of Health and Human Services, and they outline risks by age-group populations. A Guide to Clinical Preventive Services, also published by the DHHS, provides information for providers concerning burden of suffering, screening test accuracy, and efficiency of prevention for a number of illnesses associated with high morbidity and mortality.

Collecting data:
The nurse must determine a patient's risk for developing diseases or illnesses based on a multitude of factors; again, Neuman framework outlines those areas that the nurse should consider and investigate when assessing a patient's risk. The first step in any patient interview process, of course, is the detailed patient history. The information that the patient history provides for the nurse is indispensable; therefore, the nurse should attempt to elicit as much information as possible during the history-taking process, including information about the patient's family life, social life, and psychological well-being. In addition to the comprehensive history, the nurse should also expect to gain information about risk factors from the physical examination of the patient. Once the nurse has developed a risk profile for the patient based on this information, he or she can proceed to the next step in the prevention process.

Determining risk:
Typically, when trying to identify the amount of risk, the first step is hazard identification. Essentially what this means is that the adversity of the outcome (whether the risk is associated with chemical exposure, alcohol consumption, cigarette smoking, or any other risky behavior or situation) is determined based on supportive information; for example, the lifetime risk of developing emphysema in individuals with a 40 pack-year smoking history. The next step is the "dose-response analysis," the aim of which is to determine the correlation between the amount of exposure and the degree of adversity. Exposure assessment and quantification, the third step, aims to determine the probable amount of exposure that each individual within the population will receive.

Health impact assessment:
Health impact assessment is a method of assessing the potential effects of a health policy or health program on the overall health of the population targeted by the policy or program. The purpose of health impact assessment is to maximize the benefits of health programs (in addition, of course, to minimizing the negative impact that the program may potentially have). There are typically 5 steps involved in the health impact assessment project; these steps include a screening process to ensure that the program is necessary or beneficial; scoping, which determines which population(s) will be impacted by the program; identification and assessment of all potential health impacts if the program is mandated; decision making and

recommendations based on the assessment of potential impact; and evaluation and monitoring, which continues throughout the life of the program.

Risk reduction

Objectives

In 1990, the DHHS published a study entitled Healthy People 2000, in which they identified age-related and population-related risk factors. Objectives were also stated in the form of goals to be attained by the year 2000. (Note: new goals have been set for the year 2010 and can be found at http://www.healthypeople.gov.) These goals are as follows: first, to increase the overall life span for Americans; second, to reduce disparities in health across American populations; and third, to make preventive medicine services available to all Americans.

Preventive care recommendations

The USPSTF has provided preventive care recommendations based on populations that are divided by age. The age group populations were created with the idea that individuals within these age groups tend to be in similar stages of development, and share similar behavior and relationship patterns. Of course these are only guidelines, because every patient is different, but a group of adolescents tends to share more risk factors than does a group composed of a newborn, an adolescent, and an octogenarian. Based on this idea, the USPSTF created preventive guidelines for the following groups: children up to 10 years of age, people 11 to 24 years of age, people 25 to 64 years of age, people older than 65 years of age, and, as a separate risk population, pregnant women.

Lifestyle modification

<u>Birth to 10-year age group:</u>
Leading causes of death: For the birth to 10-year age group, the US Preventive Services Task Force has assembled a list of the 5 leading causes of death. The number 1 cause of death in this age group is actually a group of conditions that arise in the time period surrounding birth (the "perinatal period"). There are a number of conditions that arise surrounding birth that are fatal, including placental problems (premature separation, abruption), umbilical cord problems (cord prolapse, nuchal cord, single umbilical artery), infections (chorioamnionitis, congenital pneumonia), trauma during the birthing process (nerve damage, intracranial hemorrhage), and hemolytic disease of the newborn. The second leading cause of death is attributed to congenital defects, including tetralogy of Fallot, transposition of the great arteries, spina bifida, and anencephaly. Other leading causes of death include sudden infant death syndrome (SIDS), motor vehicle injuries, and other unintentional injuries.

Screening tests: The US Preventive Services Task Force issued a list of screening tests that are recommended for the birth to 10-year population; these screening tests were determined to be of importance based on the risks associated with this age group. Recommended screening includes height and weight measurements, which can be compared to published age-specific height and weight charts to determine whether the child is in an acceptable range. Blood pressure testing is also recommended. Vision testing is advised for children over the age of 3 (though it may be necessary in younger children if serious vision problems are suspected). In addition to these screening tests, a number of tests are recommended for all children soon after birth; these include hemoglobinopathy screening, phenylalanine level, and thyroid hormone levels (thyroxine and thyroid-stimulating hormone).

Injury prevention: Injury prevention counseling is a strong recommendation for the birth to 10-year age group, owing to the fact that motor vehicle accidents and other unintentional accidents are leading causes of death for this population. Children (and their parents) should be advised to use car safety seats until the age of 5 (this is subject to state law, however, as some states require the use of booster seats until a certain height or age is reached). After the age of 5, standard safety belts should always be used. When biking, skating, or skateboarding, a helmet should always be worn; these activities should not take place in the street. Parents should be advised to become CPR certified. They should also be advised to keep drugs, poisons, guns and other weapons, and matches out of the reach of children; to install smoke detectors and plan an escape route in the event of fire; and to make sure that stairs, windows, and pools are safe for children.

Immunizations: There are a number of immunizations that are recommended for children in the birth to 10-year age group; it is important that parents are informed of these immunizations and know at what age each should be administered. The diphtheria-tetanus-pertussis series of immunizations (DTP) are administered in 5 doses, to be given between the ages of 2 months and 6 years; the recommended progression is one dose at 2 months, followed by a dose at 4 months, 6 months, between 12 and 18 months, and again between the ages of 4 and 6 years. The oral poliovirus vaccine (OPV) is also given in 5 doses, with the same recommended progression as the DTP series. The measles-mumps-rubella vaccine (MMR) is given twice; once between the ages of 12 and 15 months, and again between 4 and 6 years of age. The H. influenzae type B vaccine is given at 2 and 4 months and again between 12 and 15 months, and the varicella vaccine between 12 and 18 months.

<u>11 to 24-year age population:</u>
Leading causes of death: The list of the top 5 leading causes of death in the 11 to 24-year age population differs significantly from the leading causes of death in the birth to 10-year age population. Leading the list for 11 to 24 year olds are deaths caused by either motor vehicle accidents or other unintentional accidents. Second on the list is homicide, followed by suicide as the third leading cause of death. The fourth leading cause of death in the 11 to 24-year age population is cancer; the most

common fatal cancers in this age group include leukemia (acute lymphocytic leukemia and acute myeloid leukemia), brain tumors (medulloblastoma, astrocytoma, and brainstem glioma), rhabdomyosarcoma, neuroblastoma, Wilm tumor, Ewing sarcoma, and Hodgkin lymphoma. The fifth leading cause of death in this age population is due to general heart diseases, which may include cardiomyopathies and faulty valves.

Screening tests: For the 11 to 24-year age population, the US Preventive Services Task Force recommends continued height and weight measurements, in addition to continued blood pressure readings. A Papanicolaou test (Pap smear) is recommended for sexually active females; if the sexual history is unknown or questionable, Pap smears should be performed for women 18 years of age and older. Sexually active individuals within this age group should also be screened for chlamydia. Immunization records should be verified in children older than 12 years of age; if the immunization history is not available, a rubella titer should be ordered.

Counseling: Individuals in the 11 to 24-year age group should be provided counseling in the following areas: injury prevention, substance use, sexual behavior, diet and exercise, and dental health. Regarding injury prevention, these individuals should be advised about the use of seat belts and helmets. Counseling about the dangers of drug, alcohol, and tobacco use is also important. This age group should be educated regarding safe sex practices and sexually transmitted disease prevention, including abstinence, condoms, and other contraceptive devices. Education should also be provided concerning the importance of a balanced diet (avoiding too much fat and cholesterol, eating a variety of grains, fruits, and vegetables, limiting sugar intake) and regular exercise. The clinician may also advise that the individual schedule regular dental checkups, and brush and floss on a daily basis.

Immunizations: For the 11 to 24-year age population, tetanus and diphtheria booster immunizations are recommended between the ages of 11 and 16 years. If the individual has not previously been immunized against the hepatitis B virus, it is recommended that he or she be immunized during this time. This immunization is administered in a series of 3, with 1 shot during the initial visit, the next shot 1 month later, and the third shot 6 months after the initial shot. If the patient did not receive his or her second MMR dose (which should have been administered between the ages of 4 and 6 years), it is advised that they be provided with the second dose between the ages of 11 and 12. If the child is susceptible to chicken pox (having not had the disease yet, and having not been previously immunized), he or she should be immunized between the ages of 11 and 12 as well.

25 to 64-year age population:

Leading causes of death: In the 25 to 64-year age population, the leading cause of death is cancer. For adult women, the leading causes of cancer deaths are lung cancer, breast cancer, colorectal cancer, pancreatic cancer, and ovarian cancer. For adult men, the leading causes of cancer deaths are lung cancer, prostate cancer, colorectal cancer, pancreatic cancer, and liver cancer. The next leading cause of death in this age group is heart disease (coronary artery disease, congestive heart failure, acute myocardial infarction), followed by motor vehicle accidents and other unintentional accidents. The fourth leading cause of death in adults age 25 to 64 is infection with HIV and its complications. Suicides and homicides account for the fifth leading cause of death.

Screening tests: Height, weight, and blood pressure measurements are again recommended as part of the screening process. Yearly total blood cholesterol testing is recommended as well, beginning at age 25 for men, and at age 45 for women. For sexually active women, a Papanicolaou test is recommended at least every 3 years; those with previously abnormal Pap smears may be advised to have this test done yearly or twice yearly, depending on the situation. Starting at the age of 50, both men and women should have yearly fecal occult blood testing, as well as a sigmoidoscopy. Yearly breast examination and mammogram is advised for women beginning at age 50 as well. Women of childbearing age should be questioned about their vaccination history; if the history of rubella vaccination is unclear or unknown, a rubella titer should be drawn.

Counseling: For the 25 to 64-year age population, counseling should be available or provided in the following areas: substance use, diet and exercise, injury prevention, and sexual behavior. Regarding substance abuse, the patient should be commended for not smoking, or, if the patient does smoke, he or she should be advised to stop smoking. The clinician should provide the smoker with some smoking cessation tips. The patient should also be advised of the ill effects of excessive alcohol use, as well as the dangers of drinking and driving. The importance of a proper, balanced diet and regular physical activity should be stressed as well. Injury prevention includes advising the patient to wear a safety belt, keep weapons in a safe place, and check smoke detectors regularly. Ways to prevent sexually transmitted disease and pregnancy can also be discussed during an intervention.

<u>Population older than 65 years of age:</u>

Leading causes of death: For adults older than 65 years of age, heart disease is the leading cause of death. In fact, heart disease is the number 1 cause of death overall in the United States. Heart disease is actually a general term for a group of diseases including cardiomyopathy, cardiovascular disease (which includes atherosclerosis and coronary artery disease), ischemic heart disease, heart failure, valvular heart disease, and hypertensive heart disease. Cancer is the second leading cause of death, with the top 3 offenders being lung cancer, breast cancer, and colorectal cancer. Cerebrovascular disease, or stroke, is the third leading cause, and is followed by or chronic obstructive pulmonary disease (COPD) as number four. The fifth leading cause of death in adults older than 65 years of age is pneumonia and influenza.

Screening tests: For adults older than 65 years of age, there are, of course, the all-important blood pressure, height, and weight measurements. Yearly fecal occult blood testing and sigmoidoscopy are also part of the screening process in this population. For women aged 65 to 69, yearly mammograms and clinical breast exams are also advised. Papanicolaou testing may or may not be necessary; this is dependent on whether past results have been consistently normal or not. If previous tests have been consistently normal, the Pap smear may be discontinued after the age of 65 (assuming that the patient is not engaging in risky sexual behavior). Adults 65 years of age and older should also have yearly vision and hearing testing as well.

Counseling: Recommended counseling for the population older than 65 is largely similar to that of the 25 to 64-year age population (advice regarding smoking cessation, excess alcohol abuse, diet and exercise, and sexual behavior). However, some additions should be noted regarding injury prevention, as this age group is at greater risk for injury. The standard counseling regarding seat belts, helmets, and smoke detectors is recommended; the clinician should also advise family members of the patient to become CPR certified in case of emergency. The patient (and his or her family members) should be counseled regarding fall prevention (confining the patient to one floor of the house, making sure that the stairs are free of clutter, placing hand rails in the bathroom).

Similarities with birth to age 10 population: When reading through the screening and counseling information recommended for these 2 age populations, you may notice that there are quite a few similarities between them. In many cases, individuals in both of these age groups must rely on another individual to provide care because they are not capable of caring for themselves. For this reason, it is suggested that the caretakers for both children and elderly persons are certified in CPR. Also, because both young children and elderly persons are sensitive to temperature, and because they are susceptible to infection and do not heal as quickly, it is recommended that the hot water heater is set so that it may not exceed 120 degrees. Because young children and elderly persons are both immunocompromised to a degree and, again, are susceptible to infection, you will notice that infection is a leading cause of death for both age populations.

Pregnant women:

First visit: The list of screening tests recommended for a pregnant woman's first visit to a clinician is somewhat lengthy. Blood pressure and weight measurements should be taken, of course. The pregnant woman's hemoglobin and hematocrit should be tested to make sure that she is not anemic, and that her baby is not being starved of oxygen and vital nutrients. A hepatitis B surface antigen test should be done to make sure that the mother has been immunized. An RPR/VRDL test should be done to detect syphilis, and if the woman is younger than 25 years of age, a chlamydia screen should also be done. Blood typing and antibody screening are also important, as well as rubella titers. Tests that may be offered, but are not required, include HIV, amniocentesis, and hemoglobinopathy screening.

Follow-up visits: When the pregnant woman is seen for a follow-up visit, blood pressure should be measured. It is important to measure the blood pressure at every visit, and to keep a close eye on it; pregnancy-induced hypertension (or preeclampsia) is a serious complication. A urine specimen should also be collected between 12 and 16 weeks; the urine should be cultured to determine whether bacteria are present. During follow-up visits, amniocentesis may again be offered to the mother; she is not required to consent to this procedure, which can identify genetic abnormalities in the fetus. Serum alpha-fetoprotein testing may also be offered; high levels of the protein have been associated with an increased risk of neural tube defects such as spina bifida. These tests are generally recommended for women older than 35 years of age, as advanced maternal age is a risk factor for certain genetic diseases.

Counseling couples:
In some situations, the clinician may find him or herself counseling a patient to stop smoking, eat healthier, and begin an exercise routine, because the patient has developed a number of health problems related to these areas. The clinician may find the patient receptive, but notices that there is no change in behavior from one visit to the next. In this case, it may be beneficial for the clinician to speak to the patient and his or her spouse. Perhaps the patient has good intentions, but has a spouse that enables him or her, or is not supportive of their lifestyle change, and so the patient does not change. By speaking to both the patient and the spouse together, the clinician may be able to get both to realize the importance of changing their habits. By committing to a change together, they may have a greater chance of succeeding.

Disease Prevention

Chemoprophylaxis
Chemoprophylaxis refers to the administration of a drug or other pharmaceutical treatment with the intention of preventing disease or infection. The initiation of chemoprophylaxis treatment may be recommended by a clinician, although the patient can refuse treatment. These recommendations may be based on age populations that are determined to be at greater risk. It is important for the clinician (and the patient) to weigh the risks and benefits of chemoprophylaxis. Examples of chemoprophylaxis include treatment for exposed individuals during outbreaks of influenza type A and influenza type B; hepatitis B immunization for health care workers, babies born to positive mothers, and individuals who have had sexual contact with a positive person; prophylactic rabies treatment for individuals who have been bitten by an animal suspected to have rabies; and rifampin prophylaxis for individuals who have been exposed to tuberculosis.

Hepatitis A
A vaccine is available for the hepatitis A virus, and should be administered to those individuals who are deemed to be at high risk of contracting the disease. Individuals

who are planning to travel to or have recently traveled to an area where hepatitis A is endemic (including Africa, South America, Mexico, and Eastern Europe) should be immunized against the virus. Other high-risk populations include drug abusers, homosexual men, and individuals who work in areas where they may come into contact with infected individuals (such as health care workers and child care workers). Those in the military should also be immunized in the event that they are stationed in an endemic country. Hepatitis A outbreaks may also occur in the food service industry when an individual does not wash his or her hands and then prepares food. In these cases, immunization is recommended for anyone who may have been exposed.

Pender's Health Promotion Model

Pender developed the Health Promotion Model in an effort to educate nurses and other clinicians about the psychosocial aspects of health promotion behavior. Her model theorizes that an individual's tendency toward health-promoting behavior is affected by his or her previous behavior, as well as his or her inherited and acquired behavioral characteristics. The individual will commit to changing his or her behavior if he or she values the benefits gained from doing so; conversely, if the individual perceives barriers in achieving these benefits, commitment may waver, and behavior modification may be abandoned. An important barrier between current behavior and behavior modification is whether the individual believes that he or she actually can accomplish an effective change in behavior with expected results.

In the Health Promotion Model, Pender proposes a number of other factors that may influence an individual's behavior modification. For example, the HPM proposes that if the individual perceives/believes that he or she is able to effectively change his or her behavior, the individual will have fewer barriers in achieving the change or changes. When the individual perceives him or herself as being effective, he or she will likely develop a positive attitude toward the behavior, which will in turn increase the individual's level of commitment. An increase in the level of commitment, then, will result in more positive results over time. The HPM also theorizes that an individual will be more willing to commit to a behavior change if a significant other values or engages in the modified behavior. Positive support from friends and family also increases the chance that the individual will remain committed.

Special needs across the lifespan

Pediatric patients

<u>Tailoring the interview process:</u>
Conducting a history and physical examination on a pediatric patient has its challenges; however, there are things that the nurse practitioner can do to make

sure that the process is as smooth and painless as possible for everyone involved. In most cases, one or more of the child's family members will be present; this will help the child to feel comfortable, but the interviewer should also strive to make sure that the child is as relaxed as possible. Speaking slowly and directly to the child, making eye contact, and getting down to the child's level are all ways to help the child feel more comfortable. Ask only one question at a time, and allow the child and his or her guardians to ask questions throughout the interview. Ask the child some questions that are not related to his or her illness; this will help establish some rapport and trust with the child.

Normal vital signs:

When evaluating the vital signs of children, it is important to take the age of the child into account, for what is normal for a child of 2 years may not be considered normal for a child of 12. Because children grow so rapidly in such a short period of time, these numbers will change rapidly as well. For a newborn baby, the normal heart rate is between 100 and 170 bpm, the normal respiratory rate is between 30 and 80 respirations per minute, and the normal blood pressure is 73/55. For a 6-month-old child, the normal ranges are 90 to 130, 24 to 36, and 80/53, respectively. Normal vitals for a 1-year-old are 90 to 130, 20 to 40, and 90/56; a 3-year-old 80 to 120, 20 to 30, and 92/55; a 6-year-old 70 to 110, 16 to 22, and 96/57; and a 10-year-old 60 to 100, 16 to 20, and 100/60.

Laboratory testing:

Because children have a much smaller volume of blood than do adults, it is often difficult to collect adequate samples for laboratory testing. Certain laboratory tests require a specific volume of blood. Historically, many tests were difficult to perform on pediatric blood samples because of inadequate sample size. Now, many laboratory tests have been modified so that smaller volumes of blood can be tested. It is helpful to know the minimum volume of blood that is required for each test to avoid having to redraw the patient; posting a list of minimum volumes for each test as a reference is a good idea. It is also important to remember that small samples should be drawn using small Microtainer tubes, because these tubes contain an adjusted amount of anticoagulant; drawing small samples into normal adult tubes (containing a larger amount of anticoagulant) can interfere with test results.

Phlebotomy:

Children, and neonates especially, are not particularly receptive to the idea of having blood drawn (though neither are most adults). There are a few things to keep in mind to make the process go as smoothly as possible. First, remember that children have much smaller veins than adults; the use of a smaller-gauge butterfly needle helps keep the phlebotomist from sticking the needle all the way through the vein, and they are easier to guide. They also look a little less intimidating to the child. Have the child turn his head away, and tell him that he will feel a little pinch before sliding the needle in. Rewarding the child afterward is a good idea. Now, when it comes to neonates and infants, the heel stick is the best (and recommended) way to obtain blood. Because the blood is typically collected one or two drops at a time, it is important to mix the blood continuously in the tube so that it does not clot, and a redraw is avoided.

Fluid requirements:
Because children are smaller than adults, and thus have a smaller blood volume, it is necessary to modify the amount of intravenous fluids that the child receives. Calculation of the amount of fluids required is based on the weight of the child in kilograms and the child's daily caloric requirements. For the first 10 kg of weight, 100 calories are required per kg; thus, a 10 kg child requires 1,000 calories (10 kg x 100 calories). 50 cal/kg/day are required for the next 10 kg, and 20 cal/kg/day are required for each kg above 20. Once the child's daily caloric needs are calculated, the fluid needs can be calculated. For a child with acute illness, intravenous fluids must provide a minimum of 20% of the overall daily caloric needs. Knowing that D5 saline provides 200 calories per 1,000 mL, an equation can be used to calculate the child's daily minimum fluid requirements.

Adult patients

Because each individual patient is exposed to different stressors that can affect the aging process, it is important to consider that some patients may experience adverse health problems, while other patients of the same age may not be affected. As individuals age, the amount of wear on the body, as well as the chance of pathology, increases; just remember that this does not happen at the same rate for every person. Factors affecting the aging process include proper nutrition (or the lack thereof), level of physical activity, smoking, alcohol consumption, environmental or occupational exposures, and socioeconomic standing. Also, remember that as an individual ages, a disease or problem with one organ or organ system will have a marked effect on other systems, because the body is not able to compensate as it once was. Symptoms may not even be noticeable until other functions begin to decline.

Illness presentation in older adults:
There are 3 major factors that influence how an illness will present in an older patient. These factors, either alone or in combination with one another, have the potential to make an ordinarily standard clinical presentation confusing for the clinician. The first of these factors is underreporting of illness or the symptoms associated with illness. There are a number of reasons that illnesses are not reported: the patient may fear hospitalization or institutionalization, or loss of control, or the patient may be convinced that there really is no problem. Another factor is the pattern of distribution of illness; this affects presentation because there are a number of diseases and problems that are prevalent among older adults, including congestive heart failure, arthritis, osteoporosis, and pneumonia. The last factor is an altered response to illness; this can make diagnosis and treatment very

difficult because symptoms may be exaggerated by other problems, or they may be nonexistent.

Pneumonia: Pneumonia, when it presents in a young, otherwise healthy adult, has a pretty standard presentation, and is not a terribly complicated diagnosis to make. The patient with pneumonia will be febrile and diaphoretic, and will complain of chills, fatigue, and difficulty breathing. The patient will produce sputum while coughing, and the sputum may be bloody. Chest pain, headache, and body aches are also common complaints. In the older patient, however, many of these symptoms may be either blunted or absent. The individual may complain of a general, nonspecific ill feeling (malaise), along with loss of appetite and weight loss. Confusion may also result because of a lack of cerebral perfusion. Tachypnea and tachycardia are common. The patient may or may not be febrile, and may or may not have a productive cough.

Iatrogenic illness:

An iatrogenic illness is defined as any illness or symptoms that occur as a result of treatment. Of course, treatment is administered with the intent to make the patient better, not worse, but sometimes treatments do have adverse effects; aging adults are especially at risk of developing an iatrogenic illness. Individuals with multisystem diseases or failures, those who take multiple medications, and those who tend toward atypical disease presentation are especially at risk. The longer a patient remains hospitalized, the more likely he or she is to develop an iatrogenic illness as well. Common iatrogenic illnesses include urinary and fecal incontinence, decubital ulcers (bedsores), muscle wasting, drug reactions, electrolyte imbalance, fluid imbalance, and even heart failure. Nosocomial (hospital-acquired) infections may also be considered iatrogenic; pneumonia and wound infections are common nosocomial infections in the older adult.

Acute confusion:

Acute confusion is a serious problem regarding aging patients, and becomes a greater risk the longer the patient remains in the hospital. The development of acute confusion in the aging patient leads to a greater risk of placement in a long-term care facility, such as hospice care or a nursing home, and also has a fairly high risk of mortality. Certain patients, when admitted, are already considered to be at risk for developing acute confusion; this includes patients older than 80 years of age, those already suffering from dementia, and those with preexisting illnesses and comorbidities. Other factors, occurring during hospitalization, may also contribute, including immobility, certain medications, infections, fluid overload, and electrolyte imbalance.

MASTER rules for rational drug therapy:

Although drugs are often very useful and effective in treating illnesses, there is a point when it becomes dangerous to the patient. Drug resistance, drug interactions, and drug intolerances are all common problems, especially among elderly patients, because an iatrogenic illness can develop. For these reasons, it is important to limit drugs to only those that are absolutely necessary. To help you decide whether a drug should be used or not, remember the MASTER rules. M is for minimizing the number of drugs a patient is taking. A is for considering alternate treatments that may be as or more effective than using a drug. S is for start low and increase slowly. Only give the patient the minimum amount, and be careful when increasing doses. T is for titration of drugs; tailor the amount given over time to the individual patient. E is for education of the patient about the drugs he or she is taking. R is for regular reviewing of drugs and doses.

Pressure ulcers:

A pressure ulcer, also known as a bedsore or a decubitus ulcer, is a very common complication in older patients; the incidence of pressure ulcers increases with the length of the patient's hospital stay. A patient who is immobile throughout the hospital stay is at an even greater risk of developing these ulcers. A patient who remains in bed without moving is placing pressure on the skin; this pressure is greatest in the areas of the body where the skin is overlying a bony prominence (the sacrum, ischial tuberosities, and heels are the most common sites for pressure ulcers). When the pressure exerted on the skin becomes greater than the capillary hydrostatic pressure, blood is unable to flow to that area. When the tissue is denied blood, it becomes ischemic. Edema and tissue death (necrosis) follow; these wounds are extremely susceptible to infection. Debridement of the dead tissue is often necessary before healing can begin.

Nurse Practitioner/Patient Relationship

Cultural competence and spiritual awareness

Cultural sensitivity

Loosely defined, cultural sensitivity refers to the ability and willingness of an individual to learn about and accept individuals who belong to different cultural groups. To understand cultural sensitivity, it helps to know what, exactly, culture is. Culture is defined as a way of life of a group of people who are united by a common language, and who share beliefs and behaviors. Nurses and other health care professionals must be culturally sensitive because they will encounter patients of various cultures, and it is important to be aware of what is acceptable to the patient. Transcultural nursing is the idea that the nurse should be knowledgeable about

Culturally competent health care:
Cultural sensitivity is an important attribute for nurses and other clinicians to possess; ignorance of other cultural beliefs can lead to alienation of the patient, which will obviously compromise the therapeutic relationship and the overall healing process. A nurse who is culturally sensitive, moreover, does not make assumptions about cultures based on broad generalizations and stereotypes. Although there may be characteristics that seem to apply to a specific culture as a whole, it is important for the nurse to remember that each person has his or her own beliefs and attitudes, regardless of cultural differences. A nurse who practices culturally competent health care is attentive and intuitive, and is able to recognize how the patient is feeling based on the patient's behavior, even if the behavior is unexpected.

Stereotype and generalization:
Stereotypes and generalizations are both detrimental to cultural sensitivity and awareness. A stereotype is defined as an oversimplified conception, opinion, or image that is based on the assumption that there are attributes that are shared between all members of another group of individuals. A generalization is defined as a broad conclusion that is based on the statistics of a small group within a population, where the said small group does not sufficiently represent the entire population. An individual who stereotypes another individual or group is indicating that he or she will not make any effort to learn about that particular individual or group, while an individual who makes a generalization may be amenable if provided more information regarding the other individual or group.

Cultural competency

8 hurdles to maintaining cultural competency:

In a study by Luckmann (1999), 8 hurdles to maintaining cultural competency were identified. These hurdles are the most significant problems that occur within the nurse-patient relationship, impeding the formation of a therapeutic relationship. It is important that the nurse be aware of these hurdles, because awareness is necessary in order for the nurse to begin the process of overcoming the hurdles. The 8 major hurdles as identified by Luckmann are as follows:

1. Lack of knowledge.
2. Fear and disgust.
3. Racism.
4. Bias and ethnocentrism.
5. Stereotyping.
6. Ritualistic behavior.
7. Language barriers.
8. Differences in perceptions and expectations.

Cultural competence model:

Campinha-Bacote et al developed a model for cultural competence; the model contains 5 components that shape the nurse's level of cultural competence. The components of the model are as follows:

1. Cultural awareness: The nurse should examine his or her own cultural beliefs and ideas, and identify any possible biases that he or she may have towards other cultures.
2. Cultural knowledge: The nurse should gather information about other cultural groups and seek to understand their beliefs and practices.
3. Cultural skill: The nurse should possess the ability to perform a cultural assessment of the patient, including a culturally based physical assessment.
4. Cultural encounter: The nurse should seek to interact with and engage patients of other cultural groups in an effort to reduce bias and increase cultural sensitivity and awareness.
5. Cultural desire: The nurse should have an interest in and a willingness to learn about other cultures so that he or she can increase cultural knowledge.

Increasing cultural knowledge:

Even the most prepared, educated nurse may at some point be required to treat a patient who belongs to a cultural group about which the nurse has little to no knowledge. In these cases, the nurse should seek to learn as much as possible about the culture in an effort to provide the patient with the best possible care. There are various resources available to the nurse who wishes to expand his or her cultural knowledge base. Journals include the International Journal of Nursing Studies, the International Nursing Review, the Journal of Cultural Diversity, and the Journal of Multicultural Nursing. Internet resources include Ethnomed (http://www.ethnomed.org) and the Foundation of Nursing Studies (http://www.fons.org), as well as information on cross-cultural healthcare (http://www.diversityrx.org).

Giger and Davidhizar cultural assessment model

Giger and Davidhizar developed a cultural assessment model to provide the nurse with a framework for assessing culturally diverse patients. The components of the model are as follows:

1. Communication: It is very important that the nurse determine the patient's preferred method of communication, as well as the patient's style of communication.
2. Space: Different cultures have different ideas about how much space is appropriate; it is important that the nurse understand the patient's spatial boundaries.
3. Social organization: Familial organization and responsibility differs between cultures.
4. Time: This is another variable that differs greatly between cultural groups. The nurse should understand that the patient may have a different concept of timing.
5. Environmental control: An individual's spiritual (and cultural) beliefs greatly affect the amount of control a patient feels he or she has over a situation and its outcome.
6. Biological variations: Some illnesses are more common in certain cultural groups than in others.

Cultural awareness

Cultural awareness assessment tool:

The cultural awareness assessment tool was developed as a way for nurses and other health care workers to gauge their own cultural awareness and sensitivity. The assessment tool is a 17-question quiz in which nurses ask themselves questions about cultural awareness. The nurse has the option of answering "always," "sometimes," or "never"; 3 points are received for each "always," 2 for each "sometimes," and 1 for each "never." The higher the nurse's score on the assessment tool, the greater his or her level of cultural awareness. Examples of statements included on the assessment tool include "I recognize the cultural differences between members of the same culture," "I have a high level of knowledge about the beliefs and customs of at least 2 different cultures," and "I know the limits of my communication skills with patients from other cultures."

Communication:

Communication is a vital part of the nurse-patient relationship; of course, as any nurse knows, establishing open communication can be difficult with any patient, even if the patient and the nurse share similar beliefs and belong to the same cultural group. When the nurse is treating a patient of another culture, especially if there is a language barrier, communication can be frustrating for both the patient and the nurse. The nurse must exercise patience when communicating, and should explore different methods of communication if one does not seem to be working. It is important that the nurse always keep in mind that the goal is to provide the best treatment possible for the patient, and that education of the patient is paramount to recovery.

Cultural awareness checklist:

Seibert et al (2002) published a cultural sensitivity and awareness checklist in the journal of medical ethics. The checklist was developed to aid clinicians in the care of patients of other cultures.

1. Identify the patient's preferred method of communication.
2. Identify language barriers and list ways to overcome them.
3. Identify the patient's culture, and make an effort to learn about the culture.
4. Ensure that the patient and the patient's family understand the situation.
5. Identify the patient's spiritual and/or religious beliefs, and contact appropriate services.
6. Determine if the patient and his or her family trust the caregivers.
7. Evaluate the patient's perceptions of his or her situation, including treatment and recovery. If the patient has misconceptions, work to correct them.
8. Determine whether the patient has any specific dietary requirements.
9. Administer patient assessments, and be alert to inaccuracies in patient comprehension.
10. Identify any biases held by the caregiver, and be aware of them.

Therapeutic communication

Therapeutic communication

Communication is important in establishing a good nurse-patient relationship. Therapeutic communication is any exchange between a health care worker and a patient; however, the goal of therapeutic communication is to foster interactions with the patient in which the patient grows and moves towards his or her treatment goals. It is important that the nurse is understanding of the fears and feelings of the patient, and can ease the patient's worries through open communication. The nurse should be available for support, and should provide any information the patient needs. The nurse should also provide feedback along the way, creating an environment where the patient feels comfortable asking questions. The patient needs to know that the nurse is listening, and that his or her concerns and ideas are being heard. These elements help establish therapeutic communication between the nurse and the patient.

Communication tools:

Patient-centered listening: Active listening on the part of the nurse (and on the part of the patient, as well) is an important part of the therapeutic communication process. For the nurse, this is referred to as "patient-centered" listening. It is important that the nurse not just hear but understand what the patient is saying, and it is important that the patient knows that the nurse is listening. When interacting with the patient, the nurse should allow the patient to do more of the talking; this, in addition to maintaining eye contact and using affirmative nonverbal communication (e.g., nodding), shows the patient that he or she is respected. The nurse should remember to keep his or her focus on the patient. By showing the patient that he or she is respected and valued, the nurse establishes the groundwork for effective therapeutic communication.

Asking questions: When communicating with a patient in an effort to establish a good nurse-patient relationship, the nurse will have to ask the patient questions. At the beginning of the nurse-patient relationship, it is best to ask the patient broad, open-ended questions. This is best for the patient, as he or she may not feel comfortable disclosing certain information; it is also helpful for the nurse, because he or she can determine the level of comfort and rapport that exists based on the patient's answers. As the relationship progresses, the nurse may ask the patient more specific questions, depending on the patient's own comfort level.

Restating: When the nurse is interviewing the patient, there are a number of ways in which he or she can make the patient feel more comfortable, and assure the patient that he or she is being heard. Eye contact and affirmative, receptive nonverbal communication is important. Another important technique is restating; to use this technique, the nurse should restate part of the patient's last comment before asking the next question. For example, the patient has described to the nurse that he has been experiencing dull, constant headaches for the past week that become more painful at night. The nurse's next question may be "You say that the pain becomes more severe at night. Is it associated with any specific activity, such as lying down?" By restating some of the patient's previous statement, the nurse shows that he or she is listening to the patient, and taking his answers seriously.

Clarification: When being interviewed, the patient may not always be able to express him or herself clearly; maybe he or she is frightened, or embarrassed, or just overwhelmed at the situation, and this is to be expected. When the nurse senses that the patient is having a hard time explaining something, he or she may ask the patient for clarification. The best way to do this is to ask the patient more specific questions, so that more specific answers can be given. The patient may be vague in his or her answers, especially because he or she is not sure what information is important to the nurse, and what information is not. By asking specific questions, the nurse is better able to understand the patient, and the patient has a better idea what the nurse needs to know. The nurse should always ask questions if he or she does not understand something the patient has said.

Reflection: Reflection is somewhat similar to restating, in that part of the purpose of the technique is to demonstrate to the patient that the nurse is listening to what he or she is saying. Reflection refers to an understanding of the patient's feelings, in addition to an understanding of what he or she is saying. When a nurse employs reflection as a communicative technique, he or she is paying attention not only to the patient's words, but also to the patient's actions and affect. The nurse can then ask the patient about his or her feelings regarding the discussion. This demonstrates to the patient that the nurse is understanding of and interested in the patient, and that the nurse is empathetic. It is important that the nurse and patient are comfortable enough with each other to reflect on feelings before the nurse attempts to use reflection as a technique so as not to make the patient uncomfortable.

Focusing: The nurse walks a fine line when attempting to establish a relationship with his or her patient; there must be mutual respect and understanding, and the patient must feel comfortable communicating with the nurse. The nurse must be able to gather important information from the patient without being brusque or demanding. Some patients may be nervous and talkative, and may want to talk about other topics in an effort to avoid discussing the issue or issues at hand. The nurse may find it necessary to focus the patient on specific areas of discussion; this should be done tactfully, so as not to make the patient feel that he or she is not important. Questions such as "do you mind if I ask you a few questions about how you are feeling about the current situation?" or "is there anything specific you would like to discuss regarding your illness?" are appropriate.

Theme identification: As the nurse has more opportunities to communicate with the patient, he or she may notice that the patient seems to be more interested in talking about some things than others, or more concerned with certain things than others. Active listening and engagement help the nurse to be more perceptive and identify specific things that are important to the patient. This process is called "theme identification"; by identifying these areas of importance, the nurse can better understand the patient's concerns. Asking the patient about these concerns ("You have mentioned being interested in alternatives to surgery, are you worried about having to undergo surgery?") shows the patient that he or she is being taken seriously, and gives him or her the opportunity to discuss specific fears and concerns more freely.

Informing and suggesting: Informing is a communicative technique whereby the nurse shares facts and information with the patient; it is important that the nurse conveys this information in such a way that the patient does not feel that he or she is being given advice by the nurse. A nurse informing a patient about something is considered to be part of the process of patient education, and the patient should be aware that the nurse is providing him or her with facts, not opinions. Suggesting, on the other hand, is more of an advice-giving technique; the nurse may provide the patient with alternative options, in addition to offering his or her opinion about which options are best for the patient.

Silence:

Although therapeutic communication is focused on active interaction between the nurse and the patient, silence can be an important part of the therapeutic relationship. In some cases, silence can be beneficial to the relationship. For example, if the patient is extremely talkative, silence on the part of the nurse can indicate to the patient that the nurse is listening and taking him or her seriously. In this case, silence is welcomed by the patient. At certain times during communication, silence can be effective, especially if it is meant to provide the patient an opportunity to reflect. If the patient is quiet, depressed, or made uncomfortable by prolonged silence, then silence on the part of the nurse could be detrimental to the relationship.

Humor:

Humor is something that almost anyone will respond to, and is an asset in various situations. Although the hospital is not typically seen as a humorous setting, humor may have a place in certain situations. Humor can be used to ease anxiety, tension, and worry, and to take the patient's mind off of an otherwise unpleasant situation. Through humor, the nurse can help the patient feel more comfortable; it sends the message that the nurse is approachable, a human being. However, the nurse must be careful, and only use humor in situations where he or she is sure that the patient will not be offended; what is funny to one person is not always funny to another.

Resistance:

Resistance from the patient is a serious roadblock in the nurse-patient relationship, and stalls therapeutic communication. There are several reasons why a patient may become resistant to communication with the nurse:

1. The patient feels that the nurse became familiar too quickly, or probed too deeply into the patient's feelings too quickly.
2. The nurse has not presented him or herself as a good role model for the patient.
3. The patient feels that there is a lack of respect from the nurse.
4. The patient does not feel comfortable communicating with the nurse because of either intentional or unintentional nonverbal cues from the nurse (no eye contact, for example).
5. The patient feels that he or she may gain something by not engaging in a therapeutic relationship with the nurse; this is sometimes called secondary gain, an example being that a patient wishes to remain in the hospital because he is homeless, and he does not want to improve himself and be discharged.

Transference:

Transference is a situation in which the patient projects feelings and attitudes towards the nurse that he or she has towards another individual (usually an authority figure) in his or her life. For example, if the nurse reminds a patient of his mother, with whom he has a poor relationship, he may treat the nurse as he would treat his mother. This is an unconscious reaction on the part of the patient, and can severely impede the therapeutic communication between the nurse and the patient. If the nurse suspects that he or she is being transferred upon by the patient, he or she must resolve the situation before the therapeutic relationship can resume.

Types of transference: Transference typically manifests in one of two ways: hostile transference or dependent reaction transference. Hostile transference may be expressed by the patient in various ways. If the patient is outwardly hostile, he or she may be uncooperative and negative; he or she may also be critical of the nurse, and challenge the nurse's decisions, or he or she may just ignore the nurse completely. If the patient internalizes his or her hostility, the nurse may see this as depression. Dependent reaction transference is much different in that the patient sees the nurse as all-knowing and all-important, and assumes a pattern of submission and dependence; in these cases, the patient depends on the nurse for everything, and the nurse may quickly become overwhelmed with demands.

Violations of boundaries

When the nurse invests time and effort into forming a therapeutic relationship with the patient, it is expected that he or she will be concerned about the well-being of the patient, and that he or she will have feelings for the patient, especially if he or she has been caring for the patient for an extended time. There are boundaries, however, and the following violate those boundaries:

1. The patient treats the nurse to lunch or vice versa.
2. The nurse accepts gifts or tips from the patient.
3. The nurse shares personal information with the patient.
4. The nurse arranges a meeting with the patient that is unrelated to treatment.
5. The nurse visits the patient at odd hours, or neglects other patients because he or she is spending too much time with one patient.

<u>Types of boundary violations:</u>
There are various ways in which the nurse-patient relationship can be violated; most of them are obvious, but some of them may not be, especially if the nurse is naïve. It is important that the nurse not violate any boundaries of his or her relationship with the patient, and therefore the nurse should familiarize him or herself with the types of boundaries that exist in the nurse-patient relationship:

1. Role boundaries: The nurse should perform his or her duties as a nurse, and nothing else.
2. Time boundaries: The nurse should not visit the patient at 3 AM if there is no therapeutic reason.
3. Place and space boundaries.
4. Money boundaries.
5. Gift and service boundaries: The nurse should not accept any gifts from the patient.

6. Clothing boundaries: The nurse should dress professionally and appropriately.
7. Language boundaries: The nurse should not use offensive language.
8. Self-disclosure boundaries.
9. Post-discharge social boundaries.
10. Physical contact boundaries.

Teaching and coaching

ACNP as an educator

The ACNP's role as an educator spans 2 major groups: patients and their families, and colleagues. The ACNP is required to educate patients about their illnesses and diseases; because patients may not possess much medical knowledge, it is important that the clinician provide information that is easily understandable. A properly educated patient is much better equipped to take care of him or herself, and can recognize potential health problems; the same applies to family members on whom the patient may rely for care. The ACNP can provide this education through a meeting with the patient and his or her family, in which treatment options and other information are discussed. Supplemental books, pamphlets, and videos are also helpful. Concerning colleague education, the ACNP may present information at rounds and conferences; he or she may also assume the role of preceptor for nursing students.

Andragogy

Andragogy (which comes from the Greek for "man-leading") is defined as the process of engaging adults in the learning process. A study conducted by Malcolm Knowles states that there are 2 basic conditions that are necessary for the education of adults. The first condition is that the educator must facilitate a climate of collaboration; in other words, the student-adult must not feel that the educator is "superior" and the student himself "inferior." There must be a mutual respect, and the student-adult must be able to trust the educator. The second condition is that the student-adult must have an active role in the learning process; he or she should be included in the needs assessment process, as well as in self-evaluation.

Knowles's assumptions of adult teaching:
In his study on adult learning, Knowles identified some of the basic assumptions that the educator can make regarding the adult learner. The first assumption is that as individuals grow and mature intellectually, we are able to direct ourselves, instead of being dependent on the directions given to us by others. The second assumption is that each individual establishes his or her own self-identity based on unique personal experiences. These experiences (and mistakes) help the individual to establish a learning process. The third assumption is that an individual's readiness to learn is based on his or her social role; in other words, an individual is

more willing and ready to learn things that directly apply to his or her job or role in life. The fourth assumption is that adults want to be able to apply knowledge immediately; this is sometimes called "problem-based learning," as opposed to traditional content-based learning.

Techniques: Knowles includes several general techniques for teaching adults as part of his study of andragogy. These techniques directly correlate to Knowles' assumptions of adult teaching; once the assumptions are understood, the teaching-learning techniques should be obvious. The first general technique is for the educator to teach adult learners based on their own past experiences. The second technique is the use of problem-based or problem-oriented learning activities, such as case studies or role-playing situational activities. The third technique is for the educator to share the responsibility of teaching with the learners, giving each learner an active role in the educational process. Adult learners should also be given an active role in evaluations. The fourth technique, aimed at keeping the adult learner interested, is to employ a variety of learning techniques and teaching strategies.

Learning theories

There are, traditionally, 3 basic learning theories: the behaviorist theory, the cognitive theory, and the social cognitive (or constructive) theory. The behaviorist theory is based on the assumption that learning is a modification of behavior based on conditioning (behavior reinforcement). Positive reinforcement is seen as a powerful moderator of learning and behavior modification. The cognitive theory is based on the idea that learning is motivated by the need for certain knowledge, and not through a change in behavior. Under the cognitive theory, an individual will be motivated to learn only the things that he or she feels are necessary to accomplish his or her life goals. The social cognitive theory is based on the idea that an individual will be more likely to modify his or her behavior if he or she has a role model to emulate.

Patient education

The Joint Commission (1994) states that "the goal of educating the patient and family is to improve patient health outcomes by promoting recovery, speeding return to function, promoting health behavior, and appropriately involving the patient in his or her own health care decisions."

<u>Needs assessment:</u>
The needs assessment is a tool used by clinicians to determine what behaviors and information the patient needs to be educated about. Once the clinician has determined what the patient's specific needs are, he or she can begin to teach the patient and the patient's family the necessary behavior modifications and information. For the ACNP, it is important to weed out the nonessential information,

because the acute care environment does not allow time for this, and the nonessential information will detract from the information that is important for the patient's recovery.

Questions: When the ACNP conducts a patient needs assessment, he or she should find out as much information as possible regarding what the patient needs to know, as well as the best way to educate the patient so that the teaching-learning process is a success. There are a number of questions that should be answered during the patient needs assessment:

1. What information does the patient already know?
2. Has the patient/family had any previous experience with this particular health issue?
3. Does the patient have any cultural beliefs that may impact his or her behavior modification?
4. What is the patient's preferred learning style?
5. Can the patient read?
6. What resources are available for use in the teaching-learning process?
7. What are the teaching and learning preferences of the ACNP?
8. What method should be used to evaluate behavior modification?
9. What will motivate the patient to change his or her behavior?
10. Are there any barriers to educating this patient?

Assessment of literacy: Before the ACNP can begin teaching the patient, he or she must formulate a teaching strategy that is appropriate for the patient. The ACNP cannot formulate a teaching strategy until he or she is familiar with the patient's literacy level. There are several available tests that the ACNP can use to evaluate the patient's literacy level. Once of these tests is the Wide Range Achievement Test (WRAT), in which the patient is given a list of words to read aloud, until he or she has made 10 mistakes in pronunciation. The patient's reading grade level is then determined by the number of words he or she has pronounced correctly.

Assessments of health and medical literacy: It is important, in addition to establishing a base literacy level, for the ACNP to establish the patient's medical literacy level; this gives the ACNP a better understanding of what the patient does know, and what the patient needs to know, about health care. The Rapid Estimate of Adult Literacy in Medicine (REALM) test is somewhat similar in style to the WRAT test; the patient is given a list of medical-related words and asked to read them. The patient's literacy score is based on the number of words he or she can pronounce. The Test for Functional Health Literacy in Adults (TOFLA) is a more comprehensive test; in addition to measuring medical literacy, it assesses the patient's medical reading comprehension and understanding of numerical values related to medicine.

<u>Motivating patients:</u>
It can be difficult for the ACNP to motivate the patient to take an active role in his or her treatment and recovery; the patient is in the hospital, sick, and probably already

overwhelmed. There are several ways in which the ACNP can motivate the patient to learn without adding to the burden. The use of visual aids is a great way to motivate the patient and hold his or her attention and interest. Rewards and praise are also great motivators; if the patient does not have much of a support system at home, this is especially important. The patient will be more likely to learn when he or she wants to know something, so it is important for the ACNP to respond to all of the patient's questions fully and in a timely manner. Teach the material to the patient beginning with easy material first, and then progressing to complex. This ensures that the patient can achieve his or her goals, which is a great motivator.

Evaluation:

The evaluation process is important, and it is beneficial not only to the patient, but to the educator as well. Regarding the patient, evaluation helps the patient figure out how to correct his or her behavior, and it also reinforces correct behavior modifications. Regarding the educator, the evaluation process determines whether the education provided is accurate. There are 2 ways in which adult patients can be evaluated: direct evaluation and indirect evaluation. Direct evaluation occurs when the educator directly observes the patient engaging in the modified behavior. When direct evaluation is not possible, an indirect approach is taken; in this case, the patient can be evaluated through his or her answers to written and/or oral questions.

Teaching patients with low literacy skills:

When educating a patient with low literacy skills, the ACNP must take special care to ensure that the material is presented in a way that the patient can easily understand. Because the patient may not understand them, it is not possible for the ACNP to hand the patient a bunch of pamphlets about the disease and treatment. Instead, the ACNP may have to devote more time to a discussion with the patient. The ACNP should frequently ask the patient questions as a method of evaluation to make sure that the patient understands the information. Other educational materials, such as videos, audiotapes, and pictures, may also be used to supplement discussions with the patient.

Interacting with a patient with disabilities:

It is to be expected that the ACNP will frequently encounter patients with disabilities. It is important that the ACNP is able to recognize what modifications he or she needs to make to his or her teaching strategies when addressing a patient with a disability. King and Cheatham have established a set of general guidelines for the ACNP to follow when interacting with a disabled patient. The first guideline is to maintain eye contact with the patient; it is important that the patient not feel uncomfortable, and it is important that the patient trust the caregiver. The next guideline is that, during the teaching process, the ACNP should always address the patient, not the patient's family members. The ACNP should also remember to encourage active participation from the patient, whether through spoken or written communication. The ACNP should also ask the patient if he or she requires any assistance with anything before providing that assistance. Lastly, but equally important, maintain a normal tone of voice.

Patient advocacy

Patient advocacy

Patient advocacy is defined as the process of speaking on behalf of a patient to ensure that his or her rights are protected, and that he or she is provided with necessary information and services. The nurse frequently serves as patient advocate, although physicians, social workers, and other individuals in the health care industry may act on behalf of the patient as well.

<u>ANA's definition of nursing:</u>
The ANA defines nursing as "the protection, promotion, and optimization of health and abilities, prevention of illness and injury, alleviation of suffering through the diagnosis and treatment of human response, and advocacy in the care of individuals, families, communities, and populations."

<u>Barriers to patient advocacy:</u>
Patient advocacy is often seen as a moral obligation that the nurse must fulfill, and is a rewarding part of the nurse's job; however, patient advocacy can be difficult in certain situations. One barrier to advocacy is a feeling of powerlessness on the part of the nurse; sometimes it may feel as if it is the nurse against the world, especially if the nurse has no support; lack of support in general is another barrier. A lack of knowledge of the law is another barrier; certain laws may exist, though the nurse may not be aware of them. If the nurse and his or her peers are lacking in time, communication, or motivation, advocacy will also prove difficult. Another problem that nurses frequently encounter is the risk associated with advocacy; included are disagreeing with other nurses and physicians, and lack of legal support for the advocate.

<u>Facilitators of patient advocacy:</u>
Perhaps the greatest facilitator of patient advocacy is the nurse-patient relationship; if a strong relationship exists between the nurse and the patient, the nurse will be motivated to perform the duties of advocate. If the patient and nurse have a strained or limited relationship, advocacy can be difficult. Recognizing the patient's needs is another facilitator, one that goes hand in hand with a good nurse-patient relationship. If the nurse feels a sense of responsibility and accountability on behalf of the patient, he or she is more likely to serve as a good patient advocate; conscience is a strong motivator. Another facilitator is if the physician acts as a colleague, instead of a superior; this strengthens the nurse-physician relationship, and the nurse feels that he or she can question the physician's judgment instead of constantly deferring. That being said, the greater the knowledge base and skill level of the nurse, the greater he or she will be as an advocate.

Reporting patient abuse

When a nurse notices that a patient is receiving improper treatment at the hands of another health care worker, be it another nurse, a physician, a social worker, or anyone else who contributes to patient care, he or she may be hesitant to report the improper treatment; this is especially true if the abusive health care worker holds a position of authority over the nurse. Although the nurse may feel that he or she should not report certain instances (even though he or she is aware that the patient is being maltreated), it is important that he or she is aware that this falls under the role of the patient advocate. Ensuring proper treatment of the patient is an important part of the nurse's job, and he or she should not worry about being reprimanded for reporting abuse.

Decisions in the best interest of the patient

The nurse is in a unique position when acting as a patient advocate; he or she typically has far more contact and interaction with the patient than any of the other members of the health care staff, and therefore has a greater opportunity to learn what is important to the patient. The increased contact with the patient also strengthens the nurse-patient relationship, and provides the nurse with motivation to be an advocate for the patient. In addition to paying attention to the patient's needs and desires as a basis for health-related decisions, the nurse also relies on his or her experience, as well as his or her sense of ethics, when making decisions about patient care.

Professional Role and Policy

Ethics

Ethical sensitivity and moral reasoning

Ethics and ethical decision making are an important part of the role of the ACNP. The advent of new technology, as well as the boom in medical research, means that the moral road is more difficult for the ACNP to navigate. Ethical sensitivity and moral reasoning are vital to the ethical decision-making process. Ethical sensitivity refers to an individual's awareness of the various moral aspects of a situation; because everyone has different values and moral guidelines, ethical sensitivity is different from one person to the next. Moral reasoning is a more analytical approach to an ethical dilemma; it refers to the process of examining all sides of a situation, and then determining what is the most ethical route or choice.

Values

A value is a belief possessed by an individual that has the power to motivate that individual's behavior. Values can be spiritual, cultural, or religious; an individual can formulate his or her own set of values based on education, and on his or her own life experiences. These values can then serve as a guideline for that individual's future decisions. Some values, however, may guide behaviors and decisions without the individual's awareness of their existence. The process of value clarification can help an individual uncover beliefs that may be negatively influencing behavior; once these beliefs and values have been uncovered, the individual can analyze and reevaluate them.

Utilitarian theory of ethics

The utilitarian theory of ethics (also referred to as the consequentialist theory) is based on the idea that the moral worth of an action is based on the overall utility, or goodness, of its consequence or consequences. Under the utilitarian theory, the ultimate importance of action is the pleasure and happiness that it produces. There are 2 basic types of utilitarianism: act utilitarianism, and rule utilitarianism. Under act utilitarianism, the individual will make his or her decisions based on the amount of pleasure derived; this is the moral code of the act utilitarian. Rule utilitarians, on the other hand, look at all the outcomes of following a particular rule when making an ethical decision. If the rule produces good results more often than it produces bad results, the rule utilitarian will always follow that rule, whereas the act utilitarian will make the decision based on whether following the rule will have a good outcome in that particular instance.

Deontological theory of ethics

Individuals who follow the deontological theory of ethics operate under the moral belief that ethical decisions should be made based on whether the action is right or wrong, and not on whether the consequences of the actions are right or wrong. Within the area of deontological ethics, however, there are those who believe that there are some actions, though not normally considered to be ethically right, that are justified based on the outcome; for example, lying is wrong, but if the consequence of the lie is that someone's life will be saved, then the lie may be seen as acceptable. Other deontologists (Kantian deontologists, named for Immanuel Kant) follow what is called moral absolutism, meaning that they will always base actions on whether the action is right, regardless of the consequences.

Ethics of care

The ethics of care, or the ethical theory of caring, is considered a normative ethical theory, meaning that the theory is based on what individuals should believe is right, instead of what individuals do believe is right. Normative ethical theories examine why certain actions are right or wrong, and why people believe that they are right or wrong, instead of adhering to strict rules about rightness and wrongness. The ethical theory of caring was proposed by feminists who felt that most traditional ethical theories were based on a male approach to problems; justice and impartiality were the guiding forces in ethical decisions. The ethical theory of caring addresses the issue that human relationships introduce complexities into ethical situations, and, as such, universal, impartial ethical rules are not sufficient bases for complex situations.

Virtue ethics

Virtue ethics is a branch of ethics that is much different than utilitarian ethics and deontological ethics. Instead of placing importance on rules and outcomes as a basis for ethical decision making, virtue ethics focuses on the character of the individual. The individual is reliant, then, on his or her own character as an ethical guide. An individual who follows virtue ethics can then be described based on his or her "moral character"; that is, his or her moral choices will reflect upon his or her character.

The casuistic theory

The casuistic theory of ethics is an applied ethical process in which decisions are made on a case-by-case basis using logic and reasoning. Cases can be compared with similar cases to guide ethical decisions.

Principle-based theory of ethics

Individuals who follow principle-based theory of ethics are guided by a set of rules, or principles, to make ethical decisions. The rules and principles that constitute principle-based ethics are formed using common and generally accepted moral practices and ideals. The principles are grouped into 4 general categories: respect for autonomy, beneficence, nonmaleficence, and justice. These 4 categories of principles share the following 2 characteristics: they are universal, meaning that they can be applied to all situations in all cultural groups; and they are all prima facie ("first appearance") binding, which means that they are accepted as the preferred method, although there may be situations in which the principle is trumped by a stronger moral consideration.

Principle of respect for autonomy:
Respect for autonomy is one of the four principles that constitute principle-based ethics; it means that people should recognize and respect that each individual has a right to make his or her own choices and formulate his or her own opinions. The individual will make decisions and form opinions based on his or her own guiding values and principles. There are exceptions to the principle of autonomy, however, and these occur when the individual is not capable, for whatever reason, of making his or her own decisions. In these cases (which must be evaluated with care), the respect for autonomy may be trumped in the interest of safety for the individual. Typically, the individual will have an appointed family member or caretaker who will be in charge of making decisions in the instance that the individual cannot.

Principle of beneficence:
Beneficence is a guiding principle in which an action is performed in such a way that it is beneficial to another person or persons; this is especially important in the world of health care, as the patient is and should always be viewed as a priority. Of course, this can become tricky when a clinician is caring for multiple patients at once, as is often the case; making decisions that constantly benefit one patient to the exclusion of others is a problem, and a compromise of time and resources must be reached. There are 5 basic rules of beneficence: protect the rights of others, prevent harm, remove sources of evil or harm, help individuals with disabilities, and help others in dangerous situations.

Principle of nonmalfeasance:
Nonmalfeasance, another of the 4 guiding principles of principle-based ethics, is the ethical or moral responsibility to avoid intentionally harming another individual. Intentional harm includes disabling or killing another individual, or inflicting pain upon another individual. This is another somewhat tricky principle to apply to medicine, and one can see how prima facie binding applies. For example, a patient is seen in the emergency department for appendicitis; he is in a great deal of pain, and at risk for rupture, peritonitis, and even death without prompt treatment. Surgical removal of the appendix is indicated, which introduces the patient to other risks

(scar from surgical procedure, postoperative pain, infection, even death). In cases such as this, nonmalfeasance may be trumped by the principle of beneficence, because the proposed risks are considered to be outweighed by the benefits.

Principle of justice:
Justice is an ethical principle that guides individuals to make decisions that are both fair and equal. Distributive justice is a specific theory that focuses on fair and equal treatment of others in regards to distributing goods and services; this theory of justice is easily applicable to medicine and health care. Because a clinician often has a group of patients that he or she is caring for at one time, it is important that the clinician divide supplies, time, and attention between the patients fairly. There are 5 material principles of distributive justice: 1) each person should receive an equal share of goods and/or services; 2) goods and services should be distributed to each individual according to the needs of the individual (entitlement); 3) each individual should receive goods and services according to effort and to 4) contribution and 5) merit.

Situations applying distributive justice: To understand how distributive justice applies to medicine, think about a situation in which there are 2 trauma patients in the emergency department. Both patients have lost a lot of blood and are in need of transfusion. The problem is, there are only 6 units of blood available. Who should get the blood? If one patient arrived before the other, should he be entitled? Perhaps he should, but there are other factors to consider. If he is in worse shape than the other patient (in other words, he needs the blood more urgently), than distributive justice would suggest that he should receive the blood. On the other hand, if both patients are in the same relative condition, how should the decision be made? You could look at contribution; if both patients were in a motor vehicle accident, but one was a drunk driver and the other an innocent motorist, it may be acceptable to give the blood to the innocent motorist in a situation where supplies are scarce.

Conditions for moral justification:
Because all principles of principle-based ethics are considered prima facie binding, there are many situations in which one principle will be trumped by another principle; this is especially true when applying principle-based ethics to medicine. When a clinician is faced with a decision in which either act may either benefit or potentially harm the patient, he or she must justify the act with the following 4 conditions: first, the act itself must be either morally good or morally neutral; second, the clinician is performing the act with only good intentions, even if he or she can foresee possible ill effects; third, the possible ill effect or effects cannot be prelude or means to the intended good effect; and fourth, the good effect or outcome must outweigh any possible ill effects.

Resolving ethical conflicts

In the health care setting, it is important that ethical conflicts be resolved without harming the patient or compromising care. There are several factors that will affect the course and outcome of an ethical conflict. First, the level of commitment the clinician has to the patient will determine the amount of effort put forth in resolving an ethical conflict. Second, the degree of moral certainty the clinician has will determine the approach to resolution; if the clinician feels that he or she is correct, he or she will most likely not waver in the decision. Third, the amount of time available for resolution is important; if the clinician is pressed for time, he or she will most likely come to a decision faster than if there is not a time constraint, in which case avoidance may occur. Fourth is the cost-benefit ratio; if the patient refuses to negotiate a certain point, for example, it is not worth the time to the clinician to try to influence the patient's decision.

Strategies:
There are many ways to attempt conflict resolution, some of them beneficial, some of them not. Avoidance is a strategy that is not typically considered to be beneficial to conflict resolution; when the clinician is not committed to the relationship with the patient, or if the situation is nonemergent, the clinician may ignore or deny the conflict in an effort to avoid facing it. Coercion is another strategy that does not usually end in a favorable outcome, at least for one of the parties involved. This strategy is used when the clinician feels that he or she is right, does not have time to devote to proper resolution, and has not invested time into a relationship with the patient. Accommodation is a somewhat similar strategy, albeit with less resistance, where one party concedes that the other's position is right. Compromise and collaboration are usually the best methods of resolution, and allow both sides to be heard.

Access to care

Diagnostic-related groups

Diagnostic-related groups (DRGs) were instituted in 1982 as a way to classify patients who shared similar diseases and treatments for billing purposes, under the assumption that patients who shared symptoms and/or diseases use the same amount of resources and should be billed the same amount. There are approximately 500 different DRGs, and patients are placed into specific DRGs using International Classification of Disease (ICD) codes, along with specific patient information such as sex, age, and the presence of comorbidities. By placing patients into DRGs, Medicare is able to determine how much the hospital should be reimbursed for patient care. The institution of DRGs has changed the health care system from one that was provider-driven (meaning the individual clinician determined the billable amount) into one that is payer-driven (meaning that Medicare determines reimbursement).

Patient-centered access to care

Access to care is often difficult for patients in nonemergent clinical situations. The patient may go to the emergency department and find him or herself waiting for hours and hours while people with more emergent problems are triaged ahead of them, leaving the patient both sick and frustrated. The patient may instead decide to call his or her primary care physician, only to find that he or she cannot be seen until after the weekend, leaving the patient to fend for himself. It is important for clinics, hospitals, and doctor's offices to provide patient-centered access to care. The characteristics of patient-centered care include availability of treatment for the patient, appropriateness of care, the ability of the patient to have a preference regarding care, and timeliness of care.

Organizing principles:

When developing a model for patient-centered access to care, organizational considerations are important; in fact, organization is vital to any care plan model, but it is especially important to patient-centered care. Disorganization is a big part of the reason that the focus has fallen away from patient centered care. A hectic, disorganized, understaffed hospital emergency room is not able to provide patient-centered care even in the best of circumstances. The following organizing principles are necessary for an effective patient-centered access to care model: first, effective use of clinical resources and expertise; second, the alignment of care with patient needs and preferences; and third, services provided where they are needed.

Outcomes management

Outcomes management is defined by Wojner as "the enhancement of physiologic and psychosocial patient outcomes through development and implementation of exemplary health practices and services, as driven by outcomes assessment." An alternate definition of outcomes management, as stated by Ellwood, is "a technology of patient experience designed to help patients, payers, and providers make rational medical care-related choices based on better insight into the effects of these choices on the patient's life." Although the 2 men had different definitions for outcome management, the line of thinking is the same, and that is the importance of a link between patient outcomes and quality control measures used to ensure that the best possible outcomes are arrived at as often as possible.

Key components:

Ellwood, in outlining the process for outcomes management, compiled a list of what are considered to be the 4 key components of any outcomes management initiative. The first of these components is that the outcomes management initiative should place emphasis on the formation or selection of standards that the clinicians can follow when planning interventions. The second component is that patient function should be measured, along with patient well-being, using disease-specific clinical outcomes as a gauge of progression. The third component is that clinical data and outcome data should be pooled together for others to use as a reference. The fourth component is that the information database should be analyzed by appropriate clinical decision makers.

Outcomes management quality model

Phase 1:

The outcomes management quality model has 4 separate phases. The first phase includes the identification of long-term outcomes for the patient in order to gauge the length of the time of care and to set a starting point. Another part of phase 1 is the selection of instruments to be used for the longitudinal study; in other words, what instruments are going to be used to determine the long-term care outcomes. These instruments typically assess quality of life, functional status, and patient satisfaction. Phase 1 also includes the identification of intermediate outcomes, which may include setbacks in the patient care process. The identification of variances that lead to setbacks in care (such as laboratory errors or physician errors) is also a part of phase 1. The last important part of phase 1 is the creation of a population database.

Phase 2:

Phase 2 of the outcomes management quality model includes the review of both traditional practice and existing literature. The overall purpose or goal of phase 2 of the model is the development of interdisciplinary practice standards. During phase 2, the members of the interdisciplinary team will gather to discuss and negotiate existing and proposed practice standards. The protocols, pathways, and order sets that are designed and formulated during this period are all considered to be "structured care methodologies" (SCMs). These SCMs will be used on the patient cohort population. Once the interdisciplinary team has decided on a set of SCMs for the cohort, the entire initiative can be standardized.

Phase 3:

Phase 3 of the outcomes management quality model is the actual implementation of the structured care methodologies within the patient cohort population. These newly instituted structured care methodologies become the standard of practice, and once the members of the interdisciplinary team and other pertinent staff members are educated about the new practices, data collection can be initiated. If the new practices are expensive (if they require expensive equipment and maintenance, or more supplies, or more billable hours initially), the interdisciplinary team should conduct a cost-benefit analysis, the obvious benefits being that length of stay, number of complications, and number of patient readmissions will be reduced as a result of the new practices.

Phase 4:

Phase 4, the final phase of the outcomes management quality model, involves a thorough, in-depth analysis of the interdisciplinary data that have accumulated during the course of the outcomes management initiative process. Once the data have been analyzed, the interdisciplinary team should meet to discuss whether certain practices or structured care methodologies should be revised to optimize outcomes management. If the team does identify practices that need revision, the initiative will return to phase 2. After this discussion, the interdisciplinary team should discuss any new questions or hypotheses that are related to outcomes management in order to perhaps begin another initiative.

Coordination of care

Nurse care coordination

Coordination of care is an important part of ensuring that the patient receives the best treatment possible. Nurses are a vital part of the coordination of care. Nurse care coordination is defined as actions that are initiated by the nurse and involve patients, their family members, and other members of the health care team. These actions are meant to manage and correct the way that care is administered to the patient, such as changing the sequence of actions (making sure that the patient is on the ward when the phlebotomist comes to draw labs, instead of sending the patient to CT and having the phlebotomist come back, for example) to optimize the effectiveness of patient care from the time the patient is admitted to the hospital until the time the patient is discharged.

Importance of coordination:
Good coordination of care results in safe and effective health care for the patient. By establishing an effective care coordination plan, the health care team will also make sure that each individual team member's job is easier; this contributes to greater job satisfaction, more time for patient interaction, and less room for error, which all together result in better patient care. Coordination of care is an especially important part of the role of the nurse, because nurses are often the first health care workers that the patient has any contact with, and they are also the health care workers that the patient has the most contact with, which means that they are in the best position for establishing care coordination.

Interdisciplinary team

The formation of an interdisciplinary team is an important part of the coordination of care. An interdisciplinary team consists of health care workers (physicians, nurses, social workers, and others) who specialize in different areas of medicine, and may work in different areas of the hospital; the team is formed because these health care workers, though in different specialties, share a common patient population and common patient care goals. Through the formation of the interdisciplinary team, active communication is established between the members of the team, their patients, and the patients' families. An interdisciplinary team may include, for example, a cardiologist, a cardiovascular surgeon, a coronary care unit nurse, and an ultrasound technician.

Beneficial to the patient:
The interdisciplinary team approach to care coordination is beneficial to the patient in several ways. First, the quality of patient care is improved because several different medical services are involved in the care of the patient, and each service is familiar with the patient's situation as a result of increased communication with other health care workers. The interdisciplinary team approach also allows the patient to have a more active role in his or her care because of the emphasis on communication between the patient and all the team members. When the clinicians work together, they also make better use of time spent with the patient, so that the patient is not subjected to lengthy history-taking sessions and redundant testing by unaware clinicians.

Beneficial to health care professionals:
In addition to being beneficial to the patient, the interdisciplinary team approach is also very beneficial to the nurse or health care professional. Perhaps the most significant benefit of this approach to care coordination is that it shifts the focus from acute patient care to long-term care that is prevention-centric. This has the added benefit of increasing professional satisfaction for the nurse, because he or she will feel that a difference is being made, and the reduction in stress makes the work environment more comfortable. Another benefit for the nurse is that when he or she is working in coordination with other specialties, he or she has more time to focus on his or her own specialty area without having to do extraneous, redundant work. The reduction in time spent performing unnecessary tasks means that the nurse has more time to learn new skills.

Beneficial to the nurse educator and the nursing student:
Acting as a nurse preceptor for nursing students is yet another role that the nurse is expected to perform, and this can be a difficult task for a nurse who is already strapped for time. When the nurse is a member of an interdisciplinary team, he or she will have more time to spend teaching nursing students; at the same time, the nursing student will find it easier to learn from a coordinated care system, rather than one that is hectic and confusing. The nursing student (and the nurse) will both benefit from being exposed to health care workers who specialize in other areas. The communicative environment of the interdisciplinary team will also encourage student participation.

Other approaches to patient care

In addition to the interdisciplinary team approach, there are several other recognized approaches to patient care. One of these approaches is the independent medical management approach, in which one clinician works alone (for the most part) with limited contact with and clinical input from other clinicians. Another approach is the multidisciplinary care approach, in which each health care worker involved in the patient care works independently of the others involved in the care of the patient; these health care workers do not collaborate, but rather each is assigned a specific task to perform. The third approach is consultative; in this case, the clinician assumes the majority of patient care, but may request consultations from other clinicians.

Hollnagel's contextual control model

Hollnagel's contextual control model is a method that was devised in order to assess how team behavior is affected by the level of organization and by environmental factors. Hollnagel proposed that when working together, a team has 4 specific modes of action; these 4 modes are strategic, tactical, opportunistic, and scrambled. The contextual control model states that the mode of action of a team is affected by the level of planning, as well as the nature of the surrounding environment. If the team has a high level of planning, the associated mode of action is strategic; conversely, if the mode of action is scrambled, the team will likely be reactive to and distracted by the environment, rather than operating by a set plan.

Cognitive model of nurse care coordination

The cognitive model of nurse care coordination is a guide to help nurses form an effective plan for the coordination of patient care. Nurse-patient communication, patient monitoring, task monitoring, and communication within the interdisciplinary care team are all important factors for the nurse to consider when assessing the overall situation; the nurse can gain a greater sense of awareness about the situation by examining all of these factors. Once the situation has been assessed, the nurse can develop a plan of action for him or herself and the other members of the interdisciplinary team, and the team can begin carrying out the necessary tasks. External factors that affect the development and execution of the care plan include the individual workload and the complexity of the tasks.

Modes of the nurse

There are 3 basic modes that the nurse may find him or herself in when coordinating patient care; these modes are based on the overall stress level at the time of planning. The first level is called steady-state mode; this is the mode that the nurse is in when the stress level is low to normal. The nurse does not feel overwhelmed and is able to handle tasks efficiently and effectively. The next level is called problem mode; in problem mode, the stress level is higher than the nurse may be able to handle by him or herself, and as such, he or she may find it necessary to delegate tasks to other members of the health care team. The third level, crisis mode, is a high-stress environment or situation where multiple people may be enlisted to help, as quick action is required.

Research Utilization

ACNP as a researcher

Research is an important part of patient care because medical advances made possible through research are the basis of future treatment modalities and care plans. The ACNP, as an advanced practice nurse, is in the perfect position to facilitate research and coordinate research efforts with current clinical practice. However, because the professional role of the ACNP is extensive, and because patient care is the most important part of the ACNP's role, it is difficult for the ACNP to find time to devote to research opportunities; it is especially difficult because there is no clearly defined research role for the ACNP. There are opportunities for ACNPs to work in a more research-oriented environment, and they can contribute a great deal to research efforts. ACNPs who work in clinical settings (as most do) may find it difficult to devote time to research.

Changing role:
The nurse practitioner is assuming an increasingly autonomous role as a health care provider because an emphasis is placed on the nurse practitioner being an "advanced practicc" clinician. The nurse practitioner may find him or herself managing a clinic with a high patient volume, or he or she may be considered an equal to resident physicians as far as responsibilities are concerned. Nurse practitioners find that they are given more patient-management responsibilities, and do not have time for teaching, education, and research. This can lead to the nurse practitioner making clinical decisions based on results that he or she observes in the clinical setting ("consensus-based" practice) instead of making decisions based on results gained from actual research-based practice.

Theory-practice gap

The theory-practice gap refers to the lack of communication between researchers and clinicians; while researchers are working to develop new treatments and methodologies, clinicians are busy treating patients and may not have the time to educate themselves about what is new in the research world. On the other side, the research community is probably not familiar with the clinical applications of the current methodologies. It is important for both sides to take an active role in communicating with one another in an effort to bridge the gap; active communication between researchers and clinicians can help disseminate new research ideas and methods into practice, and can educate researchers about what will and will not work in the clinical setting.

Bridging the theory-practice gap:
The theory-practice gap exists because clinicians and researchers traditionally work in 2 separate worlds; the clinical community is directly involved in patient care on a daily basis, while the research community is removed from the realm of patient care. Both communities, however, have the same goal, and that is to improve patient care and quality of life. Establishing communication and camaraderie between the 2 communities is incredibly beneficial for both sides. Training sessions in which clinicians are educated about research practices and researchers are trained about clinical practices are a good start. Facilitating research collaborations between researchers and clinicians is another great way to improve communication. Clinician-researchers can function as intermediaries between the 2 communities, and can educate others. The development of standard operating procedures or best practice guidelines for the transfer of knowledge is also important.

Resource-Based View

The Resource-Based View (RBV) is a theory first developed by economists with the purpose of determining the resources available to a firm or institution. It is an organizational study of the effectiveness of an institution as a result of the resources available to the institution. When applied to the theory-practice gap, the RBV is that the transfer of knowledge within and between organizations or institutions (in this case, between the clinical setting and the research setting) is costly and difficult, based on the fact that the capacity of the clinical community to absorb knowledge is low. To correct for this, the RBV states that available resources should be used to enhance and expand the learning and absorptive capacity of the clinical community.

Institutional Theory

Institutional Theory (IT), generally defined, is a theory based on the idea that it is difficult to develop institution-wide rules because there are individuals within the institution to whom the rules may not apply. These generalized institutional rules may not be feasible when applied to the daily practice of the individuals operating within the institution. This results in a gap between the actual rules of the organization and what is done by the individuals within; if the rules are not feasible, the individual may engage in evidence-based decision making. This gap between the rules and the shift to evidence-based decision making will make it more difficult to transfer knowledge both within the clinical community and between the research community and the clinical community.

Clinical challenging

"Clinical challenging" is defined as the questioning of a clinician by a nurse regarding the clinician's reasoning for making certain clinical decisions. The nurse has the opportunity to challenge the clinician on his or her decisions during patient rounds, when the clinician's explanation of his or her reasoning can benefit all of the members of the health care team who are present. The purpose of clinical challenging is for the clinician to employ critical thinking and critical decision making, rather than making decisions solely based on traditional treatment approaches. The critical thinking atmosphere promotes discussions about ongoing research that may be beneficial to the patient. If the clinician cannot provide an answer, he or she may search for information from recently published studies. Nurses may be hesitant to challenge clinicians on their decisions, but it is an important part of the learning process, and it is important for the promotion of research and the improvement of patient care.

Research resources available

Nurses, nurse practitioners, physicians, and other clinicians are often too busy to devote time to exploring the latest research advances, which could potentially be used to institute a change in practice that would greatly benefit patients. Reviewing literature can be a tedious and time-consuming process that just does not fit into the schedule of the busy clinician. There are ways that clinicians can find information about the latest practice changes and new guidelines; organizations like the Centers for Disease Control and Prevention (CDC), the National Institutes of Health (NIH), the National Cancer Institute (NCI), and the AACN often provide this information. These organizations review the literature and develop best practices, research-based protocols, and guidelines for clinicians to follow when instituting practice changes.

Developing a clinical study

Clinical challenging and other scientific-based questioning of clinical practice will often lead to questions about clinical care that the clinician does not have answers to. In these cases, the clinician may decide to develop a clinical study with the goal of answering the specific clinical question. When the clinician decides that he or she is interested in developing a research project, there are important steps that need to be followed, and important questions that need to be asked. First and foremost, the clinician needs to ask him or herself whether the study is feasible. In other words, can the study be accomplished in a reasonable amount of time, without enlisting the help of numerous people? The clinician also needs to understand all of the elements that must be included in the project, including the exact research methods, the importance of having informed consent from the patients involved in the study, the cost, and various other aspects.

Case study methodology

A great method of gaining information for the nurse is through case study methodology. The definition of a case study is "a systematic inquiry into an event or set of related events which aims to describe and explain the phenomenon of interest" (Bromley). The nurse, who has a great deal of interaction with the patient, will find that case studies are a great resource for information. When conducting a case study, the nurse will conduct a complete, comprehensive, in-depth interview of the patient, review the patient's medical records, and observe the patient.

Components of case study design:

When the nurse decides that he or she wishes to conduct a case study or a set of case studies for research purposes, he or she must design the case study in such a way that he or she elicits the most information possible from the study. First, the nurse must decide what research question or questions he or she aims to answer by conducting the case study. Second, the nurse must identify the proposition or propositions of the study. Third, the nurse must determine what exactly he or she wishes to analyze in the case study; that is, what components are vital to the questions that need to be answered. Fourth, the nurse must determine how he or she will link the data gathered through the case study to the proposition(s) of the study. Fifth, the nurse must develop standard criteria to interpret the findings yielded by the study.

Gathering meaning from research data

The data gathered from studies are often diverse, and it can be difficult to determine what is important and what is not. To determine whether data are meaningful, there are some strategies that the nurse can use. First, the nurse can look at the data to determine whether there are any patterns to see which data go with which. Then, the nurse should aim to increase his or her understanding of the data; this can be done by making comparisons between data sets, and by separating different variables within the data sets. Next, the nurse can inspect the data to see if there are any relationships between variables. Once the data have been examined and sorted, the nurse can assemble the data coherently by building a logical chain linking data and variables.

Practice Test

Practice Questions

1. A 40-year-old female hospitalized for severe exacerbation of asthma has been treated for 6 days with albuterol by small volume nebulizer, oral theophylline, and IV methylprednisolone. The patient's blood gases have stabilized. When discontinuing the IV steroid in preparation for discharge, the acute care nurse practitioner should order:

a. Inhaled steroid, such as Azmacort, only
b. Oral prednisone 20 mg daily for one week and then Azmacort
c Oral prednisone in decreasing doses
d. Oral prednisone in decreasing doses and inhaled steroid, such as Azmacort

2. A patient states, "This treatment is too much trouble." Which of the following is the best example of therapeutic communication?

a. "I agree with you."
b. "You think the treatment isn't helping you?"
c. "You should trust the doctor."
d. "Don't worry. Everything will be fine."

3. A patient who receives multiple transfusions with citrated blood products must be monitored closely for:

a. Hyponatremia
b. Hypomagnesemia
c. Hypokalemia
d. Hypocalcemia

4. Which of the following arterial blood gas (ABG) findings is consistent with metabolic acidosis in an adult?

a. HCO_3 <22 mEq/L and pH <7.35
b. HCO_3 >26 mEq/L and pH >7.45
c. $PaCO_2$ 35–45 mm Hg and PaO_2 ≥80 mg Hg
d. $PaCO_2$ >55 mm Hg and PaO_2 <60

5. When irrigating a wound, what wound irrigation pressure is needed to effectively cleanse the wound while avoiding trauma?

a. <4 psi
b. 20–30 psi
c. 10–15 psi
d. >15 psi

6. A patient has chest pain, dyspnea, and hypotension. A 12-lead ECG shows atrial rates of 250 with regular ventricular rates of 100. P waves are saw-toothed (referred to as F waves), QRS shape and duration (0.4 to 0.11 seconds) is normal, PR interval is hard to calculate because of F waves, and the P:QRS ratio is 2–4:1. Which of the following diagnoses fits this profile?

a. Premature atrial contraction
b. Premature junctional contraction
c. Atrial fibrillation
d. Atrial flutter

7. A 44-year-old obese woman recovering from a femoropopliteal bypass develops sudden onset of dyspnea with chest pain on inspiration, cough, and fever of 39°C. An S_4 gallop rhythm is present. The ECG shows tachycardia and nonspecific changes in ST and T waves. The most likely diagnosis is:

a. Myocardial infarction
b. Pulmonary embolism
c. Pneumonia
d. Sepsis

8. Which of the following is the correct procedure to evaluate the function of cranial nerve X (vagus)?

a. Ask the patient to protrude the tongue and move it from side to side against a tongue depressor
b. Observe patient swallowing, and place sugar or salt at back third of tongue to determine if patient can differentiate
c. Ask patient to swallow and speak, and place tongue blade on posterior tongue or pharynx to elicit gag reflex
d. Place hands on patient's shoulders and ask the patient to shrug against resistance

9. In Erikson's psychosocial model of development, which stage is typical of those entering young adulthood?

a. Identify vs role confusion
b. Initiative vs guilt
c. Ego integrity vs despair
d. Intimacy vs isolation

10. Which of the following is a violation of professional boundaries on the part of the acute care nurse practitioner?
   a. A nurse practitioner accepts a box of chocolates to be shared by all unit staff from a patient's daughter
   b. The nurse practitioner confides to the patient that he, like the patient, is getting a divorce, so he understands the patient's stress
   c. The nurse practitioner assists a patient in placing a call to his landlord so the patient can explain that he cannot pay the rent on time
   d. The nurse practitioner finds a patient crying and places his hand on the patient's shoulder

11. Using the average cost of a problem and the cost of intervention to demonstrate savings is:
   a. A cost-benefit analysis
   b. An efficacy study
   c. A product evaluation
   d. A cost-effectiveness analysis

12. A legal document that specifically designates someone to make decisions regarding medical and end-of-life care if a patient is mentally incompetent is a(n):
   a. Advance directive
   b. Do not resuscitate order
   c. Durable power of attorney
   d. General power of attorney

13. In evaluating outcomes of nutritional intervention for a patient with type 1 diabetes mellitus and fasting blood sugar of 130 mg/dL three months previously, which lab result most indicates dietary compliance?
   a. Fasting blood sugar of 106 mg/dL
   b. Hemoglobin A1C of 6.6%
   c. Hemoglobin A1C of 5.5%
   d. Fasting blood sugar of 150 mg/dL

14. Which is the most critical skill for a nurse collaborating in an interdisciplinary team?
   a. Patience
   b. Assertiveness
   c. Empathy with others
   d. Willingness to compromise

15. A 25-year-old patient with multiple fractures from an auto accident develops hypoxia, dyspnea, precordial chest pain, tachycardia, and thick milky sputum. Auscultation of the lungs shows crackles and wheezes. The patient complains of headache and has a fever of 40°C. Which of the following interventions should be done first?

a. High-flow oxygen
b. Corticosteroids (IV)
c. Vasopressors
d. Morphine

16. Because there is only one bed available but two patients in need of care, the acute care nurse practitioner recommends that one patient be transferred to another facility. The decision regarding which patient to transfer should be based on which ethical principle?

a. Nonmaleficence
b. Beneficence
c. Justice
d. Autonomy

17. An elderly patient states that all 15 family members may be provided information about her condition and treatment. The best method to ensure confidentiality is to:

a. Keep a list of the patient's family members on the patient's chart
b. Establish a password for family members to use when requesting information
c. Ask callers and visitors if they are family members
d. Ask the patient to limit the number of people who have access to her information

18. A patient is hospitalized for a myocardial infarction and exhibits increased preload, increased afterload, and decreased contractility with decreased cardiac output and increased systemic vascular resistance. BP is 84/40 and pulse 124 bpm, thready, and irregular. The patient has tachypnea, chest pain, basilar rales, and pallor. The most likely diagnosis is:

a. Cardiogenic shock
b. Pulmonary embolism
c. Heart failure
d. Atrial fibrillation

19. An HIV-positive patient has experienced a recent drop in CD4 count to 190. She has developed a fever with general malaise and abdominal pain, and examination shows hepatosplenomegaly. Differential diagnoses should include:

a. Pneumocystis jiroveci pneumonia, bacterial pneumonia, and TB
b. Toxoplasmosis, herpes encephalitis, and CNS lymphoma
c. Histoplasmosis, Mycobacterium avium complex, and bacillary peliosis
d. TB, non-Hodgkin's lymphoma, and bacillary angiomatosis

20. An 80-year-old male has had post-herpetic neuralgia for 11 months, but pain is increasingly intractable despite his taking 10 hydrocodone tablets daily. He has coronary stents in place and takes warfarin. The patient is weak, somnolent, and lethargic, and eats and sleeps poorly. Modifying his pain management should include:

a. Weaning patient from hydrocodone and starting gabapentin in slowly increasing doses
b. Discontinuing hydrocodone and starting morphine pump
c. Weaning patient from hydrocodone and starting biofeedback
d. Lowering the dose of hydrocodone and supplementing with NSAIDs

21. A 24-year-old female requires emergent treatment for benzodiazepine toxicity resulting from ingestion of large quantities of diazepam combined with alcohol and a combination of other unknown narcotic drugs. She exhibits pronounced lethargy, alterations in mental status, and hypotension. Treatment should include:

a. Naloxone
b. Flumazenil
c. Forced diuresis
d. Hemodialysis

22. When forced expiratory volume in one second (FEV_1) is markedly more reduced than the reduction in forced vital capacity (FVC), the patient is probably experiencing:

a. Restriction of maximal lung expansion
b. Airway obstruction
c. Depressed respiratory center
d. Limitation in neurological impulses to the muscles of respiration

23. Which of the following neurological disorders is characterized by ascending paralysis?

a. Myasthenia gravis
b. Limb-girdle muscular dystrophy
c. Guillain-Barré syndrome
d. Huntington's disease

24. A patient with a score of 10 on the Glasgow coma scale is classified as:

a. Comatose
b. Severe head injury
c. Moderate head injury
d. Mild head injury

25. Which of the following immunizations is recommended for adults ≥60?

a. Pneumococcal polysaccharides vaccine (PPV)
b. Hepatitis B
c. Hepatitis A
d. Herpes zoster

26. According to the ANA Nursing Code of Ethics, nurses must support a patient's autonomy and self-determination. If a 24-year old Asian female patient states a treatment preference but plans to leave the decision to family members, the nurse should:

a. Try to convince the patient to assert herself
b. Recognize that cultural values regarding individualism vary and respect the patient's right to be guided by family
c. Tell the family that the patient should be the one to make the decision
d. Ask the ethics committee to intervene

27. An 80-year-old patient has no insurance but is brought to the emergency room of a private hospital after a motor vehicle accident. The patient is hypovolemic and unstable, but the physician wants to transfer the patient. Which of the following acts should the nurse practitioner cite as a reason to stop the transfer until the patient stabilizes?

a. Health Insurance Portability and Accountability Act (HIPAA)
b. Emergency Medical Treatment and Active Labor Act (EMTALA)
c. Americans with Disabilities Act (ADA)
d. Older Americans Act (OAA)

28. A patient with bone metastasis from prostate cancer is to be treated with zoledronic acid (Reclast®, Zometa®). Which laboratory test(s) must be done prior to initiating treatment?

a. Serum creatinine/creatinine clearance
b. Blood urea nitrogen (BUN)
c. Complete blood count (CBC)
d. Electrolyte panel

29. A 26-year-old female with sickle cell disease states she has had numbness and aching in her right arm for about 24 hours and now has increased pain with fever. She states she has no appetite and feels increasingly anxious. Which type of crisis is consistent with these symptoms?

a. Hemolytic
b. Sequestrating
c. Aplastic
d. Vaso-occlusive

30. A 60-year-old patient with coronary heart disease is being evaluated for hyperlipidemia. Which of the following values would be of most concern?

a. HDL 50
b. LDL 90
c. LDL 165
d. Triglycerides 140

31. A 45-year-old male has renal calculi. He has passed one stone, but ultrasound shows multiple stones present in the urinary tract. Stone analysis shows the stone is calcium-containing. In addition to analgesia and antispasmodics, which medication is indicated?

a. Indomethacin
b. Allopurinol and Vitamin B6
c. Alpha-mercato-propionyl-glycine (aMPG) and captopril
d. Hydrochlorothiazide

32. When evaluating a patient with a pressure sore for acute changes in nutritional status, which may affect healing, which of the following tests is indicated?

a. Transferrin
b. Prealbumin
c. Albumin
d. Total protein

33. A 56-year-old female has pain and swelling of the small joints of the hands and wrist. Which test(s) should the acute care nurse practitioner order to confirm a diagnosis of rheumatoid arthritis?

a. Rheumatoid factor (RF) and anti-citrullinated protein antibody (ACPA)
b. RF and erythrocyte sedimentation rate (ESR)
c. C-reactive protein (CRP) and RF
d. Synovial fluid analysis, ESR, and CRP

34. With the National Pressure Ulcer Advisory Panel (NPUAP) staging system, a pressure ulcer that appears as an abrasion or blistered area without slough but with partial thickness skin loss is classified as:

a. Stage I
b. Stage II
c. Stage III
d. Stage IV

35. A patient has a chronic leg ulcer covered with black eschar and is to have chemical debridement with collagenase. Preparation includes:

a. Thoroughly drying the eschar and surrounding skin
b. Applying topical antibiotic
c. Scrubbing the wound with hexachlorophene
d. Cross-hatching the upper layers of the eschar

36. A 36-year-old female was injured in a fall when drunk. CT shows contusion on the left side of the brain. The patient responds lethargically to verbal commands and shows some confusion and restlessness. Vital signs: BP 154/76, pulse 68, and respirations 28. Previous records indicate her normal BP was 128/70, pulse 76, and respirations 16. The change in VS is most likely an indication of:

a. Increasing intracranial pressure
b. Stress response
c. Ethanol intoxication
d. Delirium tremens

37. When prioritizing differential diagnoses, which of the following is the highest priority for care?

a. Inability to respond verbally
b. Hypovolemia
c. Anxiety
d. Disturbed body image

38. A 75-year-old male is receiving warfarin after the insertion of an aortic stent for aortic aneurysm. The patient states he usually takes a number of vitamins and herbal preparations. Which of the following should the patient avoid?

a. St. John's wort
b. Melatonin
c. Echinacea
d. Vitamin B complex

39. Which of the following is an example of documentation that is currently on the Joint Commission's "Do Not Use" list?

a. 5 mg
b. 0.5 mg
c. 15 U
d. @

40. A 50-year-old female complains of recent bouts of palpitations, restlessness, and anxiety. Her skin is dry, and she complains of inability to stand excess heat or cold, difficulty sleeping, and constipation. Thyroid function tests indicate a decrease in thyroid-stimulating hormone (TSH) but increases in both T3 and T4. Which medication should the acute care nurse practitioner prescribe for the patient to take while the nurse arranges for a referral to an endocrinologist?

a. Levothyroxine (Synthroid®)
b. Metoprolol (Lopressor®)
c. Methimazole (Tapazole®)
d. Propylthiouracil

41. A retrospective attempt to determine the cause of an event, often a sentinel event such as an unexpected death, is:

a. T-test
b. Regression analysis
c. Tracer methodology
d. Root cause analysis

42. On admission, a patient is given a wristband that employs an embedded memory chip that contains information about the patient, such as name, allergies, and blood type. This is used as part of:

a. Radiofrequency identification (RFI)
b. Clinical decision support system (CDSS)
c. Computerized physician/provider order entry (CPOE)
d. Barcode medication administration (BCMA)

43. A 72-year-old female on Medicare is being discharged home with a healing burn on her left arm that she is unable to care for independently because of arthritis. She requires dressing changes every 3 days. She depends on public transportation and walks with difficulty. The bus stop is two blocks from her house. Her 12-year-old granddaughter lives with her. The best solution is:

a. Transferring the patient to an extended care facility
b. Providing treatment on an outpatient basis at the hospital clinic
c. Teaching the woman's 12-year-old granddaughter to do the dressing changes
d. Making a referral to a home health agency to provide in-home care

44. If all patients who develop urinary infections with urinary catheters are evaluated per urine culture and sensitivities for microbial resistance, but only those patients with clinically evident infections are included, this is an example of:

a. Information bias
b. Selection bias
c. Compliance bias
d. Admission bias

45. Which of the following is a necessary component of informed consent prior to a procedure?

a. Names of assisting staff members
b. Beginning and ending times
c. Risks and benefits of procedure
d. Facility statistics regarding procedure

46. When instituting a plan for risk management, which of the following is the primary concern in the statement of purpose?
   a. Reduction in financial risk
   b. Patient safety
   c. Decreased liability
   d. Scope of program

47. The purpose of an inferior vena cava filter is to:
   a. Provide an adjunct to anticoagulants
   b. Prevent myocardial infarction
   c. Prevent thrombus formation
   d. Prevent pulmonary embolism

48. A 42-year-old woman is receiving end-of-life care for stage IV breast cancer. She has developed a pronounced bronchial death rattle, which is very distressing to her adolescent daughter and son. Death is expected within a few hours. Which of the following treatments is most indicated?
   a. Glycopyrrolate or atropine sub-Q
   b. Morphine sulfate sub-Q
   c. Hyoscine hydrobromide (Scopolamine®) transdermal patch
   d. Oropharyngeal suctioning

49. A 28-year-old female who had gastric bypass surgery (Roux-en-Y) complains of bloating, abdominal cramping, nausea, and vomiting within minutes after eating. Her typical meal consists of a small potato, 3 ounces of meat, half a slice of white bread, half a banana, a small piece of cake, and 8 ounces of sweetened iced tea. Which of the following is indicated as an initial treatment?
   a. Acarbose to delay carbohydrate absorption
   b. Octreotide acetate to slow intestinal emptying
   c. Increased protein, reduced carbohydrates, and avoiding drinking during meals
   d. Decreased protein, increased carbohydrates, and a glass of juice or milk

50. A 68-year-old male has an asynchronous pacemaker and has been experiencing cardiac palpitations, headache, and anxiety, general malaise, pain in the jaw and chest, and unexplained weakness with pulsations evident in the neck and abdomen. The most likely cause is:
   a. Broken pacemaker wires
   b. Dislodged pacemaker wires
   c. Myocardial infarction
   d. Pacemaker syndrome

Answers and Explanations

1. D: Patients receiving oral or intravenous steroids should be prescribed oral prednisone in decreasing doses while initiating inhaled steroids. Severe episodes of asthma may occur with withdrawal of oral or IV steroids when switching to inhaled aerosol, so combining inhaled treatment with decreasing doses can help prevent adrenal suppression, which results in acute exacerbation of symptoms. Patients should use a metered-dose inhaler (MDI) with a reservoir device or a formulation with a spacing tube (such as Azmacort) and rinse the mouth thoroughly after inhaling to prevent thrush.

2. B: "You think the treatment isn't helping you?" is a verbal expression of an implied message. The topic should be explored while allowing the patient to terminate the discussion without probing: "I'd like to hear how you feel about that." Agreeing with rather than accepting and responding to the patient's statements can make it difficult for the patient to change his/her statement or opinion later. The nurse should avoid giving advice with "should" statements. Meaningless clichés, such as "Don't worry," can block effective communication.

3. D: Patients who receive multiple transfusions with citrated blood products must be carefully monitored for hypocalcemia. Calcium is important for transmitting nerve impulses and regulating muscle contraction and relaxation, including the myocardium. Calcium activates enzymes that stimulate chemical reactions and has a role in coagulation of blood. Values include:

- Normal values: 8.2 to 10.2 mg/dL.
- Hypocalcemia: <8.2 mg/dL. Critical value: <7 mg/dL.
- Hypercalcemia: >10.2 mg/dL. Critical value: >12 mg/dL.

Symptoms include tetany, tingling, seizures, altered mental status, and ventricular tachycardia. Treatment is calcium replacement and vitamin D.

4. A: HCO_3 <22 mEq/L and pH <7.35 are consistent with metabolic acidosis, which may result from severe diarrhea, starvation, DKA, kidney failure, and aspirin toxicity. Symptoms may include headache, altered consciousness, agitation, lethargy, and coma. Cardiac dysrhythmias and Kussmaul respiration are common. Other readings:

- HCO_3 >26 mEq/L and pH >7.45 are consistent with metabolic alkalosis.
- $PaCO_2$ 35–45 mm Hg and PaO_2 ≥80 mg Hg are normal adult readings.
- D. $PaCO_2$ >55 mm Hg and PaO_2 <60 are consistent with acute respiratory failure in a previously healthy adult.

5. C: Wounds should be irrigated with pressures of 10 to 15 psi. An irrigation pressure of <4 psi does not adequately cleanse a wound, and pressures >15 psi can result in trauma to the wound, interfering with healing. A mechanical irrigation device is more effective for irrigation than a bulb syringe, which delivers about ≤2

psi. A 250 mL squeeze bottle supplies about 4.5 psi, adequate for low-pressure cleaning. A 35-mL syringe with a 19-gauge needle provides about 8 psi.

6. D:

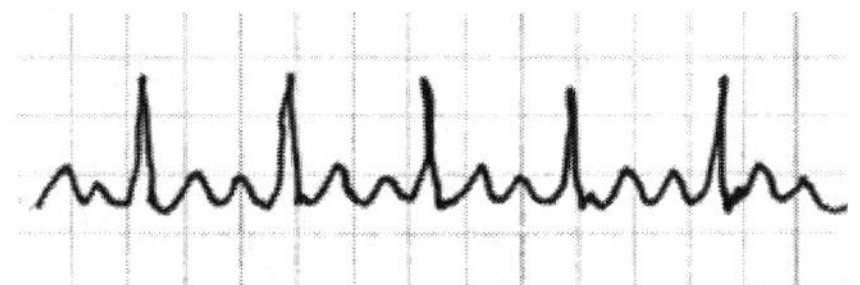

Atrial flutter (AF) occurs when the atrial rate is faster (usually 250–400 beats per minute) than the atrioventricular (AV) node conduction rate so not all of the beats are conducted into the ventricles (ventricular rate 75–150). The beats are effectively blocked at the AV node, preventing ventricular fibrillation although some extra ventricular impulses may go through. AF is caused by the same conditions that cause atrial fibrillation: coronary artery disease, valvular disease, pulmonary disease, heavy alcohol ingestion, and cardiac surgery. Treatment includes:

- Cardioversion if condition is unstable.
- Medications to slow ventricular rate and conduction through AV node: Cardizem®, Calan®.
- Medications to convert to sinus rhythm: Corvert®, Cardioquin®, Norpace®, Cordarone®.

7. B: Although symptoms of pulmonary embolism may vary widely depending on the size and location of the embolus, dyspnea, inspirational chest pain, cough, fever, S4 sound, tachycardia, and non-specific ECG changes in ST and T waves are common. Risk factors include obesity, recent surgery, history of deep vein thrombosis, and inactivity. Treatment includes oxygen, IV fluids, dobutamine for hypotension, analgesia for anxiety, and medications as indicated (digitalis, diuretic, antiarrhythmic). Intubation and mechanical ventilation may be required. Percutaneous filter may be placed in the inferior vena cava to prevent more emboli from reaching lungs.

8. C: To evaluate cranial nerve X (vagus), ask the patient to swallow and speak, observing for difficulty swallowing or hoarseness, and stimulate the back of the tongue or pharynx to elicit the gag reflex. Other examinations include:

- Cranial nerve IX (glossopharyngeal): Observe patient swallowing, and place sugar or salt at back third of tongue to determine if patient can differentiate between them
- Cranial nerve XI (spinal accessory): Place hands on patient's shoulders and ask the patient to shrug against resistance
- Cranial nerve XII (hypoglossal): Ask the patient to protrude the tongue and move it from side to side against a tongue depressor

9. D: Erikson's psychosocial development model focuses on conflicts at each stage of the lifespan and the virtue that results from finding balance in the conflict. The first 5 stages refer to infancy and childhood and the last 3 stages to adulthood:

- Intimacy vs isolation (young adulthood): Love/intimacy or lack of close relationships
- Generativity vs stagnation (middle age): Caring and achievements or stagnation
- Ego integrity vs despair (older adulthood): Acceptance and wisdom or failure to accept changes of aging/despair

10. B: The nurse should not disclose personal information, such as an impending divorce, because this establishes a social relationship that interferes with the professional role of the nurse. Small tokens of appreciation that can be shared with other staff, such as a box of chocolates, are usually acceptable (depending upon the policy of the institution), but almost any other gifts (jewelry, money, clothes) should be declined. Assisting a patient to place a phone call is not a boundary issue. Touching should be used with care, such as touching a hand or shoulder. Hugging may be misconstrued.

11. A: A cost-benefit analysis uses average cost of a problem (such as wound infections) and the cost of intervention to demonstrate savings. For example, if a surgical unit averaged 10 surgical site infections annually at an additional average cost of $27,000 each, the total annual cost would be $270,000. If the total cost for interventions (new staff person, benefits, education, and software) totals $92,000, and the goal is to reduce infections by 50% (5 X $27,000 for a total projected savings of $135,000), cost benefit is demonstrated by subtracting the intervention costs from the proposed savings ($135,000 - $92,000) for a savings of $43,000 annually.

12. C: The legal document that designates someone to make decisions regarding medical and end-of-life care if a patient is mentally incompetent is a durable power of attorney. This is a type of advance directive, which can include living wills or specific requests of the patient regarding treatment. A do not resuscitate order indicates the patient does not want resuscitative treatment for terminal illness or condition. A general power of attorney allows a designated person to make decisions for a person over broader areas, including finances.

13. C: Hemoglobin A1C of 5.5% most indicates dietary compliance. Hemoglobin AIC comprises hemoglobin A with a glucose molecule because hemoglobin holds onto excess blood glucose, so it shows the average blood glucose levels over a 3-month period and is used primarily to monitor long-term diabetic therapy. Normal value: <6% and elevation >7%. Fasting blood sugar (FBS) results can vary widely but show current serum level, so a person who stays on a diet for a few days and fasts may show a near-normal FBS for a short period even though the patient is frequently non-compliant. Normal FBS: 70–99 mg/dL.

14. D: While all of these characteristics are important for team members, central to collaboration is the willingness to compromise. In addition, members must be able to communicate clearly, which encompasses assertiveness, patience, and empathy. Teams should identify specific challenges and problems and then focus on the task of reaching a solution. Collaboration is needed in order to move nursing forward. Nurses must take an active role in gathering date for evidence-based practice to support nursing's role in health care and must share this information with other nurses and health professionals.

15. A: These symptoms are consistent with fat embolism syndrome (FES), which may cause rapid acute pulmonary edema and ARDS, so the patient should be immediately provided with high-flow oxygen. Controlled-volume ventilation with positive end-expiratory pressure (PEEP) may be indicated to prevent/treat pulmonary edema. Corticosteroids may reduce inflammation of the lungs and reduce cerebral edema. Vasopressors prevent hypotension and interstitial pulmonary edema. Morphine with a benzodiazepine may be indicated for patients who require artificial ventilation.

16. C: Justice is the ethical principle that relates to the distribution of the limited resources of healthcare benefits to the members of society. These resources must be distributed fairly. This issue may arise if there is only one bed left and two sick patients. Justice comes into play in deciding which patient should stay and which should be transported or otherwise cared for. The decision should be made according to what is best or most just for the patients and not colored by personal bias.

17. B: Care should be taken to safeguard information and provide the privacy that the patient deserves. This is accomplished through the use of required passwords when family members call or ask for information. Confidentiality is the obligation that is present in a professional-patient relationship. Nurses must protect the information they possess concerning the patient and family. The nurse must make all efforts to safeguard patient records and identification. Computerized record keeping should be done in such a way that the screen is not visible to others, and paper records must be secured.

18. A: These symptoms are consistent with cardiogenic shock. Cardiogenic shock has 3 characteristics: Increased preload, increased afterload, and decreased contractibility. Together these result in a decreased cardiac output and an increase in systemic vascular resistance (SVR) to compensate and protect vital organs. This results in an increase of afterload in the left ventricle with increased need for oxygen. As the cardiac output continues to decrease, tissue perfusion decreases, coronary artery perfusion decreases, fluid backs up, and the left ventricle fails to adequately pump the blood, resulting in pulmonary edema and right ventricular failure.

19. C: Fever, malaise, abdominal pain, and hepatosplenomegaly in an HIV-positive patient with CD4 count <200 may result from histoplasmosis, Mycobacterium avium complex, and bacillary peliosis. Fever, cough, and dyspnea may indicate Pneumocystis jiroveci pneumonia, bacterial pneumonia, and TB. Fever, headache, neck pain, and altered mental status may indicate toxoplasmosis, herpes encephalitis, and CNS lymphoma. Fever with asymmetric or unilateral lymphadenopathy may indicate TB, non-Hodgkin's lymphoma, and bacillary angiomatosis.

20. A: Post-herpetic neuralgia is a chronic pain condition that responds poorly to opioids and is better treated with anticonvulsants, such as gabapentin. Tricyclic antidepressants are also used but may have severe side effects in the elderly. Because the patient has been on high doses of hydrocodone, he may experience withdrawal with abrupt discontinuation of the drug, so the dose should be decreased by one tablet every 2 to 3 days while gabapentin is started at a low dose and slowly increased to reduce incidence of side effects. Morphine pumps and NSAIDs are usually avoided with warfarin and are often ineffective.

21. A: Benzodiazepine toxicity is treated with naloxone with co-ingestions. Flumazenil is usually contraindicated because of potential complications and is used only with pure benzodiazepine ingestion. Forced diuresis and hemodialysis have minimal effect on clearance of benzodiazepines. IV fluids are used to treat hypotension. Gastric emptying is usually avoided as it is only useful if done within one hour of ingestion. Primary care is supportive with monitoring of CNS and respiratory depression and treatment as indicated.

22. B: Airway obstruction often results in FEV_1 that is more reduced than FVC because the air is trapped and cannot be readily expelled in one second. Normally, FEV_1 is about 80% of vital capacity with most of the remaining air expelled by 3 seconds (FEV_3). Proportional reduction of both FEV_1 and FVC indicate reduced lung expansion. Depression of respiratory centers results from anesthesia or sedation. Limitation in neurological impulses results from damage to the brain or spinal cord.

23. C: Guillain-Barré syndrome (GBS) is an autoimmune disorder of the myelinated motor peripheral nervous system, often triggered by a viral gastroenteritis or Campylobacter jejuni infection. It is characterized by numbness and tingling with increasing weakness of lower extremities that often ascends to involve the arms and may become generalized, sometimes resulting in complete paralysis and inability to breathe without ventilatory support. Deep tendon reflexes are typically absent and some people experience facial weakness and ophthalmoplegia (paralysis of muscles controlling movement of eyes).

24. C: A score of 10 on the Glasgow Coma Scale (GCS) indicates a moderate head injury. GCS measures the depth and duration of coma or impaired level of consciousness and is used for postoperative/brain injury assessment. The GCS measures three parameters—best eye response, best verbal response, and best motor response—with a total possible score that ranges from 3 to 15. Injuries/conditions are classified according to the total score:

- 3–8 coma
- ≥8 severe head injury
- 9–12 moderate head injury
- 13–15 mild head injury

25. D: The herpes zoster vaccine is recommended for those ≥60 years old. A single dose of the vaccine is needed. Studies indicate that it prevents about 50% of herpes zoster cases and decreases the pain and severity of those who still develop the disease. Pneumococcal polysaccharides vaccine (PPV) is recommended for those ≥65. Hepatitis B vaccine is recommended for older adults with ESRD and hepatitis A vaccine for those at risk depending upon lifestyle (males who have sex with other males or illegal drug users) or medical condition (chronic liver disease, those receiving clotting factor concentrates).

26. B: Under the ANA Nursing Code of Ethics, autonomy and self-determination are viewed within the broad context of diverse cultures. The idea of individualism is less important in some cultures, so the nurse must respect and appreciate the patient's right to be guided by her family. Trying to convince the patient to assert herself may just lead to emotional conflict. This is not an appropriate concern for the ethics committee, as the woman is not being forced to comply with family decisions but chooses to do so.

27. B: EMTALA prohibits patient "dumping" from EDs. Stabilization of emergent conditions or active labor must be done prior to transfer, and the patient's condition should not deteriorate during transfer. HIPAA addresses the rights of the individual related to privacy of health information. ADA is civil rights legislation that provides people with disabilities, including those with mental impairment, access to employment and the community. OAA provides improved access to services for older adults and Native Americans, including community services (meals, transportation, home health care, adult day care, legal assistance, and home repair).

28. A: Because zoledronic acid may result in decreased renal function in acute renal failure, a serum creatinine and calculation of creatinine clearance should be done before every dose. Zoledronic acid is contraindicated with creatinine clearance <35 mL/min or with severe renal impairment. Additional treatments are withheld if renal deterioration occurs and not resumed until creatinine is within 10% of baseline value. Normal CC values: Adult male: 97–137 mL/min: Adult female: 88–128 mL/min. During treatment, patients should receive calcium (500 mg) and vitamin D (400 IU) supplements daily unless the patient has hypercalcemia.

29. D: These symptoms are consistent with vaso-occlusive crisis. The 4 phases of vaso-occlusive pain include:

- Prodromal: (one day prior to pain onset) Numbness, aching, paresthesia
- Initial/Infarctive: Fever, pain, anxiety, anorexia
- Established/Post-infarctive: (up to 4 or 5 days) Severe pain with inflammation, swelling, joint effusions, arthralgia
- Resolving: Decrease in pain over 24–48 hours

Bone is the most common site for vaso-occlusion, but it can occur in the abdomen, brain, chest, or organs (liver, kidneys). When extremities are involved, patients may develop dactylitis with swelling and pain in hands or feet.

30. C: The optimal LDL goal for those with CHD or equivalent risk is <100 mg/dL.

LDL cholesterol	<100 Optimal 100–129 Near optimal 130–159 Borderline high 160–189 High ≥190 Very high
Total cholesterol	<200 Optimal 200–239 Borderline high ≥240 High
HDL cholesterol	<40 Low ≥60 High
Triglycerides	<150 Normal 150–199 Borderline-high 200–499 High ≥500 Very high

31. D: Thiazides, such as hydrochlorothiazide, are indicated to increase reabsorption of calcium with calcium-containing renal calculi. Allopurinol and vitamin B6 are used with oxalate-containing stones. Alpha-mercato-propionyl-glycine (aMPG) and captopril are used with cystine-containing stones if increasing hydration and alkalinization is ineffective. Indomethacin is used with allopurinol to maintain uric acid levels. Alkalinizing agents, such as Polycitra and Allopurinol, are used with uric acid stones. Additional medications can include antibiotics if infection occurs. Some patients may require opioids, such as morphine, to control pain.

32. B: Prealbumin (transthyretin) is most commonly monitored for acute changes in nutritional status because it has a half-life of only 2–3 days:

- Normal values: 16–40 mg/dL.
- Mild deficiency: 10–15mg/dL.
- Moderate deficiency: 5–9 mg/dL.
- Severe deficiency: <5 mg/dL.

A decrease in iron stimulates the liver to produce more transferrin but also decreases production of albumin and prealbumin. Thus, transferrin levels alone are not always reliable measurements of nutritional status. Albumin has a half-life of 18–20 days, so it is sensitive to long-term protein deficiencies more than short-

term. Total protein levels can be influenced by many factors but may be monitored as part of an overall nutritional assessment.
33. A: Tests for diagnosis of rheumatoid arthritis in the presence of joint involvement of the small joints (fingers, wrists) or large joints (elbows, hips, knees) includes primarily RF and ACPA. ESR and CRP may also show elevation but are less specific. Diagnosis is usually made if 4 of 7 positive symptoms for RA are present: morning stiffness >1 hour, ≥2 involved joints with involvement of wrists, or finger joints >6 weeks, bilateral and symmetrical involvement, presence of rheumatoid nodules, joint destruction on x-ray, and positive RF or ACPA.

34. B: Stage II. NPUAP Stages include:

- Suspected deep tissue injury: Skin discolored, intact or blood blister
- Stage I: Intact skin with non-blanching reddened area
- Stage II: Abrasion or blistered area without slough but with partial-thickness skin loss
- Stage III: Deep ulcer with exposed subcutaneous tissue. Tunneling or undermining may be evident with or without slough
- Stage IV: Deep ulcer, full thickness, with necrosis into muscle, bone, tendons, and/or joints
- Unstageable: Eschar and/or slough prevents staging prior to debridement

35. D: Chemical debridement is used for chronic wounds (burns, ulcers) with necrotic tissue and eschar. However the enzymes (collagenase and papain/urea) require a moist environment, so the eschar must be cross-hatched through the upper layers before the enzyme is administered. The pH must remain between 6 and 8 to prevent inactivation. Hexachlorophene, Burrow's solution, and heavy metal ions also inactivate the enzymes. Collagenase is applied one time daily, either directly to the wound for deep wounds or to gauze packing for shallow wounds.

36. A: These VS changes are consistent with increasing intracranial pressure. Typical findings include widened pulse pressure, with rising blood pressure and depressed heart rate. Because the patient is drunk, evaluating level of consciousness can be difficult, but lethargy, confusion, and restlessness are characteristic of increasing ICP. Stress response usually results in increased BP and pulse. Ethanol intoxication usually causes hypotension, bradycardia with arrhythmias, and respiratory depression. Delirium tremens includes tremors, tachycardia, and cardiac dysrhythmias.

37. B: Hypovolemia is a physiologic need and takes priority over other needs.

1	Physiological (basic needs to sustain life—oxygen, food, fluids, sleep)	Risk for aspiration. Deficient fluid volume. Impaired spontaneous ventilation.
2	Safety and security (physiological and psychological threats)	Verbal communication impaired. Latex allergy response. Death anxiety.
3	Love/Belonging (support, caring, intimacy)	Risk for loneliness. Anxiety. Caregiver role strain.
4	Self-esteem (sense of worth, respect, independence)	Defensive coping. Disturbed body image. Post-traumatic response.
5	Self-actualization	Health-seeking behaviors. Spiritual distress.

38. A: St. John's wort may interact with antibiotics, birth control pills, antidepressants, warfarin, anticonvulsants, MAO inhibitors, antivirals, immunosuppressants, and migraine drugs. Melatonin may interact with NSAIDS, antihypertensives, steroids, and anti-anxiety medications. Echinacea may interact with immunosuppressants and steroids. Vitamin B complex is safe to take with warfarin, as it does not affect the INR; however, multivitamins with vitamin K may. If patients take a multivitamin during warfarin therapy, they should do so daily and not intermittently so that intake of vitamin K does not fluctuate. Vitamin C should be limited to 500 mg daily and vitamin E to 400 IU daily.

39. C: The abbreviation of U for units is on the "Do Not Use" list. Other prohibited abbreviations/symbols include IU; QD; QOD; MS, MSO, and MgSO4 for morphine or magnesium sulfate; trailing zeros (4.0 mg) and lack of leading zero (0.4 mg). Additional abbreviations/symbols are allowed but under consideration for future prohibition. These include <, >, @, cc, μg, and abbreviations of drug names (such as TCN for tetracycline). Using the correct word or term is always better than using an abbreviation, which may be misunderstood, especially if writing is not clear.

40. B: These symptoms are consistent with hyperthyroidism, which poses a risk of adverse cardiac events, so the patient should be placed on a β-blocker, such as Lopressor, for stabilization until further assessment by an endocrinologist. If patients are unable to take β-blockers, they may be prescribed calcium channel blockers although they may be less effective. Synthroid is used for hypothyroidism. Methimazole and propylthiouracil are both antithyroid medications, usually the

treatment of choice because of risks associated with surgery, although thyroidectomy may be done in some cases.

41. D: Root cause analysis is a retrospective attempt to determine the cause of an event. Regression analysis compares the relationship between two variables to determine if the relationship correlates. T-test is used to analyze data to determine if there is a statistically significant difference in the means of two groups. The t-test looks at two sets of things that are similar, such as exercise in women over 65 with cancer and over 65 without cancer. Tracer methodology is a method that looks at the continuum of care a patient receives from admission to post-discharge.

42. A: RFI is an automatic system for identification that employs embedded digital memory chips, with unique codes, to track patients, medical devices, medications, and staff. CDSS is an interactive software application that provides information to physicians or other healthcare providers to help with healthcare decisions. CPOE is a clinical software application that automates medication/treatment ordering, requiring that orders be typed in a standard format to avoid mistakes in ordering or interpreting orders. BCMA utilizes wireless mobile units at the point of care to scan the barcode on each unit of medication or blood component before it is dispensed.

43. D: The best solution is a referral to a home health agency to provide in-home care, as this ensures that the woman will receive skilled nursing care and be able to stay at home and supervise her granddaughter. A 12-year-old is too young for the responsibility of wound care. The patient's dependence on public transportation and difficulty walking precludes outpatient care. Home health care is a more cost-effective solution than transferring the patient to an extended care facility, which would leave the granddaughter without care. Medicare will not pay for extended hospital care for healing wounds.

44. B: This is an example of selection bias because those with catheters without clinically evident infections were excluded. The results are skewed because many patients may have subclinical infections. Information bias occurs when there are errors in classification, so an estimate of association is incorrect. Information bias may be non-differential or differential. Compliance bias occurs when adherence to protocol is inconsistent. Admission bias occurs when some groups, such as spinal cord injury patients, are omitted from the study.

45. C: Patients/family should be apprised of all reasonable risks and any complications that might be life threatening or increase morbidity as well as benefits. The American Medical Association has established guidelines for informed consent:

- Explanation of diagnosis
- Nature and reason for treatment or procedure
- Risks and benefits
- Alternative options (regardless of cost or insurance coverage)
- Risks and benefits of alternative options

- Risks and benefits of not having a treatment or procedure
- Providing informed consent is a requirement of all states

46. B: Patient safety should always be the primary concern for risk management. Reduction of financial risks and liability relate directly to patient safety. A risk management plan should include:
    - Goals: Specific and measurable
    - Program scope: Should include linkage with other programs
    - Line of authority: Beginning with the governing board and ending with employees
    - Policies: This should include confidentiality and conflict of interest.
    - Data sources and referrals: Types of measures
    - Documentation/reporting: The responsibility for reporting should be clarified and the frequency of reports
    - Activities integration
    - Evaluation of program: The method and frequency of evaluation
    - Charts/Diagrams: Flow charts, organizational charts, and diagrams

47. D:. The IVC filter is inserted, usually through the right internal jugular vein, into the inferior vena cava to prevent pulmonary emboli, especially for patients with recurrent pulmonary emboli. The filter prevents dislodged thrombi from entering the lungs. The filter may be used for patients who cannot tolerate anticoagulants or in whom they are contraindicated, such as a patient with a recent stroke. Anticoagulants should be continued with the IVC filter if possible. Some newer IVC filters are removable and may be left in for extended periods of time, such as weeks or months.

48. A:. Glycopyrrolate or atropine sub-Q has rapid onset of action (about 1 minute). Glycopyrrolate provides stronger action. Morphine sulfate may reduce respiratory distress but does not generally affect death rales. The hyoscine hydrobromide (Scopolamine®) transdermal patch has a slow onset of action (about 12 hours), so it is best used for long-term treatment. Oropharyngeal suctioning may relieve rales originating in the oropharynx but is ineffective for pooling of fluids in the bronchi.

49. C: Dumping syndrome usually responds to a change in dietary habits and is most often caused by carbohydrate intake, so increasing protein, reducing carbohydrates, and avoiding drinking fluids with meals may relieve symptoms. Acarbose is sometimes used with late-onset dumping syndrome (occurring 1 to 3 hours after eating) if other methods are ineffective. Octreotide requires injections and is used only for intractable symptoms because of adverse effects, such as diarrhea, distention, and cholelithiasis.

50. D: These symptoms are consistent with pacemaker syndrome.

Mild	Pulsations evident in neck and abdomen. Cardiac palpitations. Headache and feeling of anxiety. General malaise and unexplained weakness. Pain or "fullness" in jaw, chest.
Moderate	Increasing dyspnea on exertion with accompanying orthopnea Dizziness, vertigo, increasing confusion. Feeling of choking.
Severe	Increasing pulmonary edema with dyspnea even at rest and crackling rales. Syncope. Heart failure.

Secret Key #1 - Time is Your Greatest Enemy

Pace Yourself

Wear a watch. At the beginning of the test, check the time (or start a chronometer on your watch to count the minutes), and check the time after each passage or every few questions to make sure you are "on schedule."

If you are forced to speed up, do it efficiently. Usually one or more answer choices can be eliminated without too much difficulty. Above all, don't panic. Don't speed up and just begin guessing at random choices. By pacing yourself, and continually monitoring your progress against your watch, you will always know exactly how far ahead or behind you are with your available time. If you find that you are one minute behind on the test, don't skip one question without spending any time on it, just to catch back up. Take 15 fewer seconds on the next four questions, and after four questions you'll have caught back up. Once you catch back up, you can continue working each problem at your normal pace.

Furthermore, don't dwell on the problems that you were rushed on. If a problem was taking up too much time and you made a hurried guess, it must be difficult. The difficult questions are the ones you are most likely to miss anyway, so it isn't a big loss. It is better to end with more time than you need than to run out of time.

Lastly, sometimes it is beneficial to slow down if you are constantly getting ahead of time. You are always more likely to catch a careless mistake by working more slowly than quickly, and among very high-scoring test takers (those who are likely to have lots of time left over), careless errors affect the score more than mastery of material.

Secret Key #2 - Guessing is not Guesswork

You probably know that guessing is a good idea - unlike other standardized tests, there is no penalty for getting a wrong answer. Even if you have no idea about a question, you still have a 20-25% chance of getting it right.

Most test takers do not understand the impact that proper guessing can have on their score. Unless you score extremely high, guessing will significantly contribute to your final score.

Monkeys Take the Test

What most test takers don't realize is that to insure that 20-25% chance, you have to guess randomly. If you put 20 monkeys in a room to take this test, assuming they answered once per question and behaved themselves, on average they would get 20-25% of the questions correct. Put 20 test takers in the room, and the average will be much lower among guessed questions. Why?

1. The test writers intentionally writes deceptive answer choices that "look" right. A test taker has no idea about a question, so picks the "best looking" answer, which is often wrong. The monkey has no idea what looks good and what doesn't, so will consistently be lucky about 20-25% of the time.
2. Test takers will eliminate answer choices from the guessing pool based on a hunch or intuition. Simple but correct answers often get excluded, leaving a 0% chance of being correct. The monkey has no clue, and often gets lucky with the best choice.

This is why the process of elimination endorsed by most test courses is flawed and detrimental to your performance- test takers don't guess, they make an ignorant stab in the dark that is usually worse than random.

$5 Challenge

Let me introduce one of the most valuable ideas of this course- the $5 challenge:

You only mark your "best guess" if you are willing to bet $5 on it.
You only eliminate choices from guessing if you are willing to bet $5 on it.

Why $5? Five dollars is an amount of money that is small yet not insignificant, and can really add up fast (20 questions could cost you $100). Likewise, each answer choice on one question of the test will have a small impact on your overall score, but it can really add up to a lot of points in the end.

The process of elimination IS valuable. The following shows your chance of guessing it right:

If you eliminate this many choices:	0	1	2	3	4
Chance of getting it correct	20%	25%	33%	50%	100%

However, if you accidentally eliminate the right answer or go on a hunch for an incorrect answer, your chances drop dramatically: to 0%. By guessing among all the answer choices, you are GUARANTEED to have a shot at the right answer.

That's why the $5 test is so valuable- if you give up the advantage and safety of a pure guess, it had better be worth the risk.

What we still haven't covered is how to be sure that whatever guess you make is truly random. Here's the easiest way:

Always pick the first answer choice among those remaining.

Such a technique means that you have decided, **before you see a single test question**, exactly how you are going to guess- and since the order of choices tells you nothing about which one is correct, this guessing technique is perfectly random.

Let's try an example-

A NP encounters the following problem:

Which of the following characteristics match an arterial wound assessment done by a NP?
A: Painful, pain at rest
B: Medial aspect of lower leg
C: Increased temperature
D: Red, purple color

The test taker has a small idea about this question- he is pretty sure that the characteristic is "increased temperature," choice C, but he wouldn't bet $5 on it. He knows that the characteristic is either "painful, pain at rest" or "increased temperature," so he is willing to bet $5 on both choices B and D not being correct. Now he is down to A and C. At this point, he guesses A, since A is the first choice remaining.

The test taker is correct by choosing A, since the characteristic match would be "painful, pain at rest". He only eliminated those choices he was willing to bet money on, AND he did not let his stale memories (often things not known definitely will get mixed up in the exact opposite arrangement in one's head). He blindly chose the first remaining choice, and was rewarded with the fruits of a random guess.

This section is not meant to scare you away from making educated guesses or eliminating choices- you just need to define when a choice is worth eliminating. The $5 test, along with a pre-defined random guessing strategy, is the best way to make sure you reap all of the benefits of guessing.

Similar Answer Choices

When you have two answer choices that are direct opposites, one of them is usually the correct answer.
Example:

A. Secretes cholesterol
B. Synthesizes cholesterol

These two answer choices are very similar and fall into the same family of answer choices. A family of answer choices is when two or three answer choices are very similar.

Summary of Guessing Techniques

1. Eliminate as many choices as you can by using the $5 test. Use the common guessing strategies to help in the elimination process, but only eliminate choices that fail the $5 test.
2. Among the remaining choices, only pick your "best guess" if it passes the $5 test.
3. Otherwise, guess randomly by picking the first remaining choice that was not eliminated.

Secret Key #3 - Practice Smarter, Not Harder

Many test takers delay the test preparation process because they dread the awful amounts of practice time they think necessary to succeed on the test. We have refined an effective method that will take you only a fraction of the time.

There are a number of "obstacles" in your way to succeed. Among these are answering questions, finishing in time, and mastering test-taking strategies. All must be executed on the day of the test at peak performance, or your score will suffer. The test is a mental marathon that has a large impact on your future.

Just like a marathon runner, it is important to work your way up to the full challenge. So first you just worry about questions, and then time, and finally strategy:

Success Strategy

1. Find a good source for practice tests. You will need at least 2 practice tests.
2. If you are willing to make a larger time investment (or if you want to really "learn" the material, a time consuming but ultimately valuable endeavor), consider buying one of the better study guides on the market.
3. Take a practice test with no time constraints, with all study helps "open book." Take your time with questions and focus on applying the strategies.
4. Take a practice test with time constraints, with all guides "open book."
5. Take a final practice test with no open material and time limits

If you have time to take more practice tests, just repeat step 5. By gradually exposing yourself to the full rigors of the test environment, you will condition your mind to the stress of test day and maximize your success.

Secret Key #4 - Prepare, Don't Procrastinate

Let me state an obvious fact: if you take the test three times, you will get three different scores. This is due to the way you feel on test day, the level of preparedness you have, and, despite the test writers' claims to the contrary, some tests WILL be easier for you than others.

Since your future depends so much on your score, you should maximize your chances of success. In order to maximize the likelihood of success, you've got to prepare in advance. This means taking practice tests and spending time learning the information and test taking strategies you will need to succeed.

Since you have to pay a registration fee each time you take the test, don't take it as a "practice" test. Feel free to take sample tests on your own, but when you go to take the official test, be prepared, be focused, and do your best the first time!

Secret Key #5 - Test Yourself

Everyone knows that time is money. There is no need to spend too much of your time or too little of your time preparing for the test. You should only spend as much of your precious time preparing as is necessary for you to pass it.

Once you have taken a practice test under real conditions of time constraints, then you will know if you are ready for the test or not.

If you have scored extremely high the first time that you take the practice test, then there is not much point in spending countless hours studying. You are already there.

Benchmark your abilities by retaking practice tests and seeing how much you have improved. Once you score high enough to guarantee success, then you are ready.

If you have scored well below where you need, then knuckle down and begin studying in earnest. Check your improvement regularly through the use of practice tests under real conditions. Above all, don't worry, panic, or give up. The key is perseverance!

Then, when you go to take the test, remain confident and remember how well you did on the practice tests. If you can score high enough on a practice test, then you can do the same on the real thing.

General Strategies

The most important thing you can do is to ignore your fears and jump into the test immediately- do not be overwhelmed by any strange-sounding terms. You have to jump into the test like jumping into a pool- all at once is the easiest way.

Make Predictions

As you read and understand the question, try to guess what the answer will be. Remember that several of the answer choices are wrong, and once you begin reading them, your mind will immediately become cluttered with answer choices designed to throw you off. Your mind is typically the most focused immediately after you have read the passage and question and digested its contents. If you can, try to predict what the correct answer will be. You may be surprised at what you can predict.

Quickly scan the choices and see if your prediction is in the listed answer choices. If it is, then you can be quite confident that you have the right answer. It still won't hurt to check the other answer choices, but most of the time, you've got it!

Answer the Question

It may seem obvious to only pick answer choices that answer the question, but the test writers can create some excellent answer choices that are wrong. Don't pick an answer just because it sounds right, or you believe it to be true. It MUST answer the question. Once you've made your selection, always go back and check it against the question and make sure that you didn't misread the question, and the answer choice does answer the question posed.

Benchmark

After you read the first answer choice, decide if you think it sounds correct or not. If it doesn't, move on to the next answer choice. If it does, tentatively check that answer choice. This doesn't mean that you've definitely selected it as your answer choice, it just means that it's the best you've seen thus far. Go ahead and read the next choice. If the next choice is worse than the one you've already selected, keep going to the next answer choice. If the next choice is better than the choice you've already selected, check the new answer choice as your best guess.

The first answer choice that you select becomes your standard. Every other answer choice must be benchmarked against that standard. That choice is correct until proven otherwise by another answer choice beating it out. Once you've decided that no other answer choice seems as good, do one final check to ensure that your answer choice answers the question posed.

Valid Information

Don't discount any of the information provided in the question. Every piece of information may be necessary to determine the correct answer. None of the information in the question is there to throw you off (while the answer choices will certainly have information to throw you off). If two seemingly unrelated topics are discussed, don't ignore either. You can be confident there is a relationship, or it wouldn't be included in the question, and you are probably going to have to determine what is that relationship for the answer.

Avoid "Fact Traps"

Don't get distracted by a choice that is factually true. Your search is for the answer that answers the question. Stay focused and don't fall for an answer that is true but incorrect. Always go back to the question and make sure you're choosing an answer that actually answers the question and is not just a true statement. An answer can be factually correct, but it MUST answer the question asked. Additionally, two answers can both be seemingly correct, so be sure to read all of the answer choices, and make sure that you get the one that BEST answers the question.

Milk the Question

Some of the questions may throw you completely off. They might deal with a subject you have not been exposed to, or one that you haven't reviewed in years. While your lack of knowledge about the subject will be a hindrance, the question itself can give you many clues that will help you find the correct answer. Read the question carefully, and look for clues. Watch particularly for adjectives and nouns describing difficult terms or words that you don't recognize. Regardless of if you understand a word or not, replacing it with the synonyms used for it in the question may help you to understand what the questions are asking.

Look carefully for these descriptive synonyms (nouns) and adjectives and use them to help you understand the difficult terms. Rather than wracking your mind about specific detail information concerning a difficult term in the question, use the more general description or synonym provided to make it easier for you.

The Trap of Familiarity

Don't just choose a word because you recognize it. On difficult questions, you may not recognize a number of words in the answer choices. The test writers don't put "make-believe" words on the test; so don't think that just because you only recognize all the words in one answer choice means that answer choice must be correct. If you don't recognize words in all but one answer choices, then focus on the one that you do recognize. Is it correct? Try your best to determine if it is correct. If it does, that is great, but if it doesn't, eliminate it. Each word and answer choice you eliminate increases your chances of getting the question correct, even if you then have to guess among the unfamiliar choices.

Eliminate Answers

Eliminate choices as soon as you realize they are wrong. But be careful! Make sure you consider all of the possible answer choices. Just because one appears right, doesn't mean that the next one won't be even better! The test writers will usually put more than one good answer choice for every question, so read all of them. Don't worry if you are stuck between two that seem right. By getting down to just two remaining possible choices, your odds are now 50/50. Rather than wasting too much time, play the odds. You are guessing, but guessing wisely, because you've been able to knock out some of the answer choices that you know are wrong. If you are eliminating choices and realize that the last answer choice you are left with is also obviously wrong, don't panic. Start over and consider each choice again. There may easily be something that you missed the first time and will realize on the second pass.

Tough Questions

If you are stumped on a problem or it appears too hard or too difficult, don't waste time. Move on! Remember though, if you can quickly check for obviously incorrect answer choices, your chances of guessing correctly are greatly improved. Before you completely give up, at least try to knock out a couple of possible answers. Eliminate what you can and then guess at the remaining answer choices before moving on.

Brainstorm

If you get stuck on a difficult question, spend a few seconds quickly brainstorming. Run through the complete list of possible answer choices. Look at each choice and ask yourself, "Could this answer the question satisfactorily?" Go through each answer choice and consider it independently of the other. By systematically going through all possibilities, you may find something that you would otherwise overlook. Remember that when you get stuck, it's important to try to keep moving.

Read Carefully

Understand the problem. Read the question and answer choices carefully. Don't miss the question because you misread the terms. You have plenty of time to read each question thoroughly and make sure you understand what is being asked. Yet a happy medium must be attained, so don't waste too much time. You must read carefully, but efficiently.

Face Value

When in doubt, use common sense. Always accept the situation in the problem at face value. Don't read too much into it. These problems will not require you to make huge leaps of logic. The test writers aren't trying to throw you off with a cheap trick. If you have to go beyond creativity and make a leap of logic in order to have an answer choice answer the question, then you should look at the other answer choices. Don't overcomplicate the problem by creating theoretical relationships or explanations that will warp time or space. These are normal problems rooted in reality. It's just that the applicable relationship or explanation may not be readily apparent and you have to figure things out. Use your common sense to interpret anything that isn't clear.

Prefixes

If you're having trouble with a word in the question or answer choices, try dissecting it. Take advantage of every clue that the word might include. Prefixes and suffixes can be a huge help. Usually they allow you to determine a basic meaning. Pre- means before, post- means after, pro - is positive, de- is negative. From these prefixes and suffixes, you can get an idea of the general meaning of the word and try to put it into context. Beware though of any traps. Just because con is the opposite of pro, doesn't necessarily mean congress is the opposite of progress!

Hedge Phrases

Watch out for critical "hedge" phrases, such as likely, may, can, will often, sometimes, etc, often, almost, mostly, usually, generally, rarely, sometimes. Question writers insert these hedge phrases, to cover every possibility. Often an answer choice will be wrong simply because it leaves no room for exception.

Switchback Words

Stay alert for "switchbacks". These are the words and phrases frequently used to alert you to shifts in thought. The most common switchback word is "but". Others include although, however, nevertheless, on the other hand, even though, while, in spite of, despite, regardless of.

New Information

Correct answer choices will rarely have completely new information included. Answer choices typically are straightforward reflections of the material asked about and will directly relate to the question. If a new piece of information is included in an answer choice that doesn't even seem to relate to the topic being asked about, then that answer choice is likely incorrect. All of the information needed to answer the question is usually provided for you, and so you should not have to make guesses that are unsupported or choose answer choices that require unknown information that cannot be reasoned on its own.

Time Management

On technical questions, don't get lost on the technical terms. Don't spend too much time on any one question. If you don't know what a term means, then since you don't have a dictionary, odds are you aren't going to get much further. You should immediately recognize terms as whether or not you know them. If you don't, work with the other clues that you have, the other answer choices and terms provided, but don't waste too much time trying to figure out a difficult term.

Contextual Clues

Look for contextual clues. An answer can be right but not correct. The contextual clues will help you find the answer that is most right and is correct. Understand the context in which a phrase is stated. This will help you make important distinctions.

Don't Panic

Panicking will not answer any questions for you. Therefore, it isn't helpful. When you first see the question, if your mind goes blank, take a deep breath. Force yourself to mechanically go through the steps of solving the problem and using the strategies you've learned.

Pace Yourself

Don't get clock fever. It's easy to be overwhelmed when you're looking at a page full of questions, your mind is full of random thoughts and feeling confused, and the clock is ticking down faster than you would like. Calm down and maintain the pace that you have set for yourself. As long as you are on track by monitoring your pace, you are guaranteed to have enough time for yourself. When you get to the last few minutes of the test, it may seem like you won't have enough time left, but if you only have as many questions as you should have left at that point, then you're right on track!

Answer Selection

The best way to pick an answer choice is to eliminate all of those that are wrong, until only one is left and confirm that is the correct answer. Sometimes though, an answer choice may immediately look right. Be careful! Take a second to make sure that the other choices are not equally obvious. Don't make a hasty mistake. There are only two times that you should stop before checking other answers. First is when you are positive that the answer choice you have selected is correct. Second is when time is almost out and you have to make a quick guess!

Check Your Work

Since you will probably not know every term listed and the answer to every question, it is important that you get credit for the ones that you do know. Don't miss any questions through careless mistakes. If at all possible, try to take a second to look back over your answer selection and make sure you've selected the correct answer choice and haven't made a costly careless mistake (such as marking an answer choice that you didn't mean to mark). This quick double check should more than pay for itself in caught mistakes for the time it costs.

Beware of Directly Quoted Answers

Sometimes an answer choice will repeat word for word a portion of the question or reference section. However, beware of such exact duplication – it may be a trap! More than likely, the correct choice will paraphrase or summarize a point, rather than being exactly the same wording.